RISING FROM THE
ASHES

*My Journey to Transform Grief and
Depression into Purpose and Destiny*

IGNACIO E. LEON

RISING FROM THE
ASHES

My Journey to Transform Grief and
Depression into Purpose and Destiny

For More Information:
Fig Factor Media | figfactormedia.com

Cover Design by Marco Alvarez
Layout by LDG Juan Manuel Serna Rosales

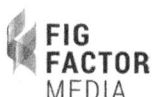

Printed in the United States of America

ISBN: 978-1-959989-82-0

To the memory of my beloved son, Alexander Estefan Leon, who left this world too soon at the age of twenty. Your absence has left an indescribable void in my heart, but your spirit continues to guide me every day.

This book is also dedicated to all those who are fighting the silent oppressor of mental illness, especially depression and grief. May it serve as a light of hope and understanding for those who feel enveloped in the darkness.

Table of Contents:

Acknowledgments

To my wife, Debra, and daughter, Ava: Your unwavering support has been the bedrock of my journey through the most challenging times. Your love and resilience have been my guiding lights, and for that, I am eternally grateful.

I would like to express my heartfelt gratitude to my dear friend and editor, Andre Faulkner, for generously dedicating her precious time and unwavering energy to assist me in editing this book. Her invaluable contributions have played a pivotal role in shaping and refining the content, making it the best it can be. I am also immensely grateful to my brother and close friend, Michael J. Leon, for his unwavering support and tireless efforts in helping me bring this book to life. His time, energy, and invaluable ideas and inspiration have been instrumental in guiding me through this incredible journey. Together, we have triumphed over challenges and created a work that truly reflects the essence of our shared experiences. Thank you, Andre and Michael, for being an integral part of this remarkable endeavor.

I extend my deepest gratitude to the friends, family, and community who have provided steadfast support and understanding. Your kindness and compassion have been instrumental in our journey of healing.

A heartfelt thank you to my former coworkers, managers, mentors, and the compassionate individuals I've encountered along the way. Your generosity and support have inspired me to give back and make a difference in the lives of those grappling with pain and loss.

May these words serve as a testament to the strength found in togetherness, guiding us to rise from the ashes, find solace in our shared experiences, and heal from the wounds of grief and mental illness.

Foreword

As I sit here, pen in hand, reflecting on the journey that led me to this moment, I am overwhelmed with a sense of gratitude and awe. It is with great honor that I write this forward for my husband, Ignacio, and his book, "Rising from the Ashes."

From the very beginning, Ignacio has been a source of inspiration and strength in my life. His unwavering love and support have carried me through the darkest of times, and it is through his own resilience and determination that he has emerged as a beacon of hope for others.

When we received the news about our son's suicide, it felt as though our world had shattered into a million pieces. The weight of uncertainty and fear threatened to consume us, but Ignacio stood tall, refusing to let despair take hold. He became a pillar of strength, for me and our daughter Ava.

In the face of adversity, Ignacio's unwavering faith and unwavering belief in our son's ability to overcome depression became a guiding light. He tirelessly researched, sought out the best resources, and advocated for our son's needs. Ignacio's love knew no bounds as he dedicated himself to understanding and supporting our son's journey towards healing.

Through his own experiences and struggles, Ignacio found the courage to share his story with others. He bared his soul, laying bare the raw emotions and challenges that come with navigating the complexities of mental health. His honesty and vulnerability have touched the hearts of many, offering solace to those who find themselves in similar situations.

"Rising from the Ashes" is a testament to Ignacio's unwavering belief in the power of resilience and the human spirit. It is a story of hope, redemption, and the unbreakable bond of family. Ignacio's words have the power to uplift, to inspire, and to ignite a flame of hope in the hearts of those who read them.

To my love Ignacio, thank you for sharing your journey with the world. Your courage, compassion, and unwavering love have touched the lives of many, including mine. Your words have the power to heal, to bring light to the darkest corners of the human experience. I am honored to stand by your side as we continue to rise from the ashes, together.

With all my love,
Debra

Prologue
January 2019

In the quiet of our bedroom, I sat with Debra, my wife, her face reflecting the gravity of the news she had just received.

"So, you're saying . . . " I paused, my voice catching with a mixture of disbelief and concern as I repeated her words, ". . . our son has bipolar disorder with manic depressive episodes?"

"Yes, Chito, that's what the therapist told me," she replied, her gaze fixed on some distant worry.

I tried to wrap my head around it. "Can you break it down for me? What does that even mean?"

She took a breath, trying to put it into words we could grasp.

"It's like extreme mood swings, Chito. When he's in a manic phase, he'll have this high energy, his thoughts might race, and he might act impulsively. But then, in the depressive phase, it's like a deep sadness, fatigue, and a feeling of hopelessness."

"So, he's going to have these really up moments and then really down ones?"

"Yeah, exactly," she nodded, her eyes searching mine for understanding.

A heavy weight settled in the room as the disbelief within me grew stronger. How could such a diagnosis align with the memories of my son, the one who had always embraced life with unbridled enthusiasm and spirit?

My vibrant and lively then eighteen-year-old son, Alexander, "Xanny" or "Xan" to us, was a source of boundless joy, the crown jewel of our lives. He epitomized love, kindness, and an eagerness to make his parents proud, bringing smiles and laughter to all who met him. From grade school to junior high, teachers marveled at his intellectual engagement, labeling him an "old soul" with wisdom beyond his years.

But as I grappled with the therapist's words and Debra's somber confirmation, one memory flashed through my mind that suddenly filled in a piece of the puzzle.

Actively involved and passionate about the performing arts since a young age, we had received a call from Xanny's theater teacher during the summer of his sophomore year in high school while he was taking an acting class. She told us about an exercise where the class was asked to delve into the spectrum of emotions an actor might need for a role. Each student was asked to express a joyous moment from that summer. As the class played out their experiences, the teacher noticed Xanny appeared to be struggling. Puzzled, she approached him.

He revealed an unsettling truth: he couldn't think of a single moment that had brought him joy. The teacher tried to offer suggestions; surely there had to be one? Xanny, she told us, had just shook his head.

Thinking back on that call, coupled with the therapist's diagnosis, gave me a glimpse into a side of Xanny I had been oblivious to, a side he had hidden so well. For a moment, I allowed myself to acknowledge the pain he might have been silently carrying. I had gone through myself what I considered a very difficult inner struggle in my teen years, defined by secret bouts of depression and months of emotional turmoil. I just figured that, with a little help, he would navigate himself through it, just like I did.

It was an unsettling moment of introspection, putting together pieces of a puzzle that unveiled a portrait of my son that was both complex and deeply human. Recognizing his struggle went far below the surface, I responded as I believed any parent would, finding strength in my resolve to help my son.

"No, this is unacceptable," I told Debra. "Xan will be fine. He's smart, his friends and family absolutely love him. He has the whole world in front of him! Everyone has ups and downs; every teenager goes through mood swings and emotional challenges.

"I'm going to talk to him. We will get this straightened out. We can get him help, do therapy, and, if necessary, add some medication. We can pray with him and for him, and he will be fine. No problem," I declared, clinging to the belief that we could pave a path forward for our son.

Despite our best efforts, we could not.

THE ESSENCE OF MY STORY: A MESSAGE OF HOPE AND HEALING

They say that the loss of a child is every parent's worst nightmare. But it goes far beyond that. It's worse. So much, much worse than you could ever imagine.

This is my story of what surviving such an incomprehensible tragedy is like. While tragic, it is a story I hope can help others embedded in the throes of profound grief—whatever loss they may be mourning—not only survive but to eventually thrive in spite of it.

My story is a testament to the possibility of healing, even from the most devastating losses.

My message is one of hope. It's an assurance that no matter how deep your wounds, there is a way to heal them. There is light beyond the darkness, peace beyond the pain, and a future beyond the grief. This story, my journey, is shared in the spirit of helping you see that possibility for yourself.

My intention is to offer a glimpse into the entire spectrum of the healing process, to paint a vivid picture of what lies beyond the immediate pain and despair. It is to show you that, regardless of the depth of your suffering, there is a path forward to a place where you can be healthy and whole again.

I want to illuminate the journey for you, not just the destination. It's a journey that acknowledges the reality of pain and grief, but also one that leads toward a brighter horizon where hope and healing reside. This is not about forgetting or negating your loss but about learning to live with it in a way that allows for growth, peace, and renewed purpose.

AFFIRMATION OF PURPOSE AND REASON

I want to affirm something crucial, something that has become a beacon of light in my journey through the darkest times. Each of us, including you who are reading this, is here for a reason. Our lives, though sometimes battered by the storms of loss and sorrow, are imbued with purpose and meaning.

This affirmation is not just a platitude; it's a fundamental truth that I've come to embrace. In the aftermath of losing my son, I questioned everything—my beliefs, my choices, the very purpose of my existence. But through this tumultuous journey, I've discovered that even in the midst of profound grief, we can find reasons to continue, to heal, and to grow.

Our purpose might not always be clear, especially when shrouded in the fog of great sorrow. But it's there, woven into the very fabric of our being. It's in the way we touch the lives of others, in the love we share, and in the unique perspectives we bring to the world. Our purpose is in the legacy we build and leave behind, influenced by those we have loved and lost.

So, I offer you this affirmation as a source of strength and encouragement: you have a purpose, a reason for being here. Your journey through grief is a part of that purpose. It shapes you, tests you, and ultimately, can lead you to a deeper understanding of yourself and the world around you.

Embracing this truth has been a pivotal part of my healing process. It has given me the strength to push back against the pain, to find moments of joy amidst sorrow, and to continue writing my story—a story that is still being crafted, with Xan's memory etched into every word.

Your story, too, continues. It's a narrative filled with potential, waiting to unfold in all its complexity and beauty. As you move forward on your journey, hold onto this affirmation of purpose and reason. Let it guide you through the challenging days and remind you of the resilience that lies within you.

Ignacio E. Leon

Chapter 1:

THAT FATEFUL DAY

Stuck

"Hey, Xanny, remember those concrete baseballs?" I exclaimed, pointing towards the large sculptures that greeted us at the entrance of the stadium.

The day was bright, filled with the promise of quality time with my teenage son, Alexander, who we affectionately called Xanny. There he stood, his height hinting at maturity yet to come, his grin infectious, and his wit sharp.

A handsome young man with light brown hair and a fair complexion, he was the embodiment of the joy and intelligence that had always defined him. However, a shadow of something unspoken, a slight weight seemed to have settled on his shoulders lately, perhaps the stress of navigating the complexities of high school and the daunting path to college.

"I remember that, dad," he responded with a chuckle, offering me a smile that seemed a bridge between the carefree laughter of his youth and the more reserved demeanor he now carried.

A smile of my own found its way to my lips as I drifted back to a day five years earlier, a day so full of laughter and shared joy that it seemed to belong to another lifetime.

That day, as we had made our way to watch the Diamondbacks take on the San Diego Padres, Xanny, a younger, lighter version of himself, was a whirlwind of twelve-year-old energy and happiness. We explored the stadium, indulging in every available delight, from hot dogs and popcorn to snapping photos and picking up souvenirs, his laughter making every moment brighter.

We came across the large concrete baseballs at the entrance. With the fearless bravado of youth, Xanny exclaimed, "I'm going to jump over them!" Encouraged by my nod, he took a running start, but instead of making the leap over, found himself awkwardly perched atop one, struggling to get down.

I went over and, with a gentle tug, helped him down. We stood there, laughing together, then embraced—a moment of pure connection.

"Remember, Xan, anytime you get stuck, just let me know, and I'll come help you out," I said, a pledge that felt as solid as the ground beneath our feet.

My mind returned to the present and as I looked at him, I suggested, "Come on, Xanny! See if you can leap over those baseballs again!"

This time he opted to simply pose in front of them rather than jump over, a compromise between then and now. But, with some gentle fatherly urging, he reluctantly agreed to give it a try. In a moment, his teenage athleticism was on display as he launched into a springy run, effortlessly cartwheeling over the ball. I captured the moment with my camera, our laughter mingling in the air, but a part of me couldn't help but wonder about the changes in him.

Since turning sixteen, Xanny had seemed different, less open, perhaps, or simply caught in the throes of adolescence. Could it be the usual teenage angst or was there something more? I recalled my own dark days at his age, the silent battles with depression, and wondered if history was repeating itself.

"It's okay," I reassured myself as we continued to our seats, my hand finding its way to his shoulder in a gesture of support. "He might be a little stuck right now, but he's got us. We're here for him, just like when he was twelve." That thought warmed me from the inside out, bolstering my resolve to be there for him, no matter what.

As we settled in to enjoy the game, my gaze lingered on Xanny, his profile etched against the backdrop of the field. In that moment, all the complexities of life seemed insignificant compared to the enduring bond between us, a bond that no challenge could ever diminish.

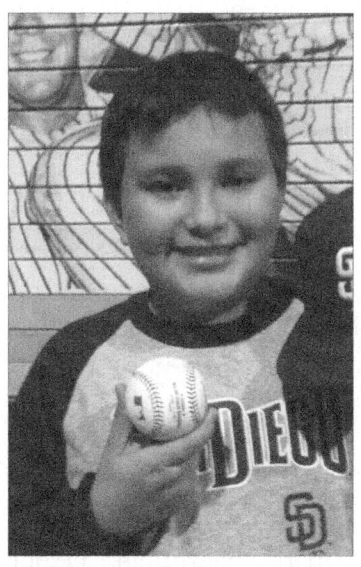 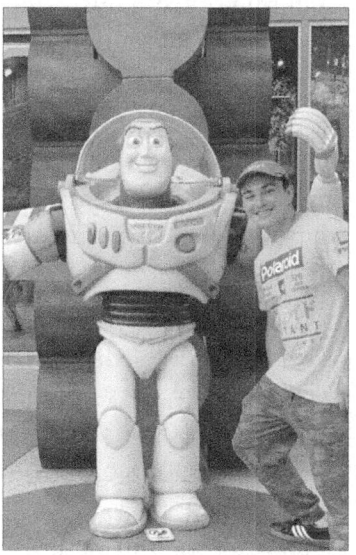

***

OCTOBER 27, 2019

"He's not answering."

The morning sun cast a deceptive glow over our friend's home in Phoenix, but the warmth it promised failed to thaw the growing unease within me.

My wife, Debra, and I had just finished a hike and were expecting to enjoy a relaxing Sunday morning with our dear friends Kent and Chervet. This moment was anything but relaxing though, as we were trying to reach our son who was hours away in Flagstaff, Arizona.

He was supposed to show up at work at 7 a.m. for his weekend college campus radio show; but his best friend, Diego, had just contacted us to let us know that Xanny never arrived. It was something that had never happened before.

Repeated calls to Alexander went unanswered, each ring a disconcerting reminder of the silence on the other end, Debra's mounting concern mirroring my own. Her eyes, once filled with the assurance of routine, now reflected the unsettling void left by our son's unresponsiveness.

"Chito, he's never missed work without a call. What if something's wrong?" Her voice trembled, the air heavy with an unspoken fear. I tried to offer reassurance, the words falling from my lips like feeble attempts to stave off the encroaching darkness.

"Debra, it could be anything. Maybe he left his phone at home, or it's on silent, or the battery died. There are countless reasons to explain this. Let's not jump to conclusions," I urged, my own voice betraying the tension beneath the surface. But despite the rationalizations, the gnawing worry persisted.

Intensified by the persistent unanswered calls, memories of our son, so full of life, echoed in the background of our conversation along with an unspoken fear, cast by the shadow of our son's diagnosis earlier that year that he suffered from bipolar disorder and manic depression.

Yet another attempt to reach him went straight to voicemail, a hollow confirmation of our escalating concern. "Maybe he's out with friends," I suggested, grasping at the frail hope that this was merely a mundane deviation from routine. Yet, with each futile call, that hope waned as dread took root.

"We can't keep waiting. What if something's happened?" Debra's eyes pleaded for action, her maternal instincts overriding the dwindling rationalizations.

I hesitated. "Let's give it a bit more time," I suggested, a desperate attempt to cling to the semblance of control.

As minutes stretched into an agonizing eternity, we tried reaching out to friends and acquaintances, sending texts that remained unanswered. The dread, an insidious presence, settled deeper within us, overshadowing the feeble attempts at optimism.

"I can't wait any longer," Debra said, gathering her things in her hands and searching for the keys. "I'm heading up there."

Her movement ignited the spark of action in the room, as I rushed into the kitchen where my keys and wallet were.

"You're not going by yourself, I'll drive. Let's go to Flagstaff."

As we headed toward the front door, there stood our dear friends, their keys and coats in hand.

"Chito, you both are way too emotional to drive right now," Kent said, his eyes somber and determined. "We'll drive."

We all breathed a collective breath and headed for the car.

The Sunday morning, once drenched in sunlight, now turned dark with the weight of our uncertainty as we embarked on a journey into the unknown. The car's engine roared to life, drowning out the unspoken fears that echoed within the confines of our shared solitude.

Hurtling down the highway, Debra and I huddled in the back seat, our phones ablaze with frantic texts and calls, desperately reaching out to anyone who might have a clue about our son's whereabouts. The situation grew increasingly dire as our efforts yielded little information.

Then, another message from Diego pierced through the chaos. "You both need to come now." The gravity of those words hung in the air, as true terror took root in our hearts.

The car became a crucible of stress, each passing moment intensifying the suffocating atmosphere. Time stretched and contorted, every minute an agonizing pulse of uncertainty. Electricity surged through our fingertips, the anticipation of what awaited us almost unbearable.

Flashbacks flooded my mind. I recalled the day Xan left for college and the ensuing weeks of parental sadness—along with a foreboding sense that when he departed, it would mark the last time he would be with us. I had brushed off the premonition then; but now, with each passing mile, it felt like my soul had sensed something my conscious mind hadn't grasped.

Please, God, I repeated like a mantra, just let him be okay. Please, God, just let him be okay.

The car screeched to a halt outside Xan's dorm building on the Flagstaff campus. In a panic, we darted out and rushed through the door, our hearts pounding, each step fueled by a mix of hope and dread, the warmth of the morning sun unable to penetrate the cold grip of fear that enveloped us.

"I need to see my son, Alexander. He didn't show up for his radio show, and he's not answering any calls," I blurted out to the attendant, my voice layered with anxiety.

The attendant, though sympathetic, insisted on protocol, saying she needed to check first before allowing us to go up to his room. This bureaucratic delay felt torturous, adding to our already heightened stress.

In the waiting area, each minute stretched into what seemed like an eternity. Our collective anxiety was palpable. Kent and Chervet did their best to hold us together as our minds raced, imagining the worst.

Impatience and worry got the better of me. I approached the attendant again, my tone firm.

"I'm going in there. I can't wait any longer," I said. But before I could take another step, the silent flashes of approaching lights caught my attention from the corner of my eye. Collectively, we turned our heads towards the ambulance as it pulled up to the building, our hearts sinking.

Debra's voice cracked as she asked, "Is that for my son? Is that for my SON?"

The attendant, now looking equally worried, tried to calm us, but her words were drowned out by the sirens.

Almost simultaneously, a police officer emerged from within the dorm building, his expression somber, eyes reflecting a sorrow too deep for words. The world seemed to stop, the ambient noises around us fading into an eerie silence. He took a deep breath, and with tears brimming in his eyes, he delivered the words that shattered our world.

"I'm sorry. He didn't make it."

The officer continued to speak, but his words were muffled, drowned out by the rushing sound in my ears, like waves crashing relentlessly against a shore. The words hit like a physical blow, sending a shockwave through my body. My knees weakened, and I felt myself falter, the ground seemingly slipping away beneath me. Debra let out a heart-wrenching cry, her hands covering her face as if to shield herself from the unbearable reality. Her cry would not stop from that moment on.

Our son, Alexander Estefan Leon, was gone.

Chapter 2:

A SOUL LAID BARE

Running in Zigzags

The car embraced the winding roads on the outskirts of Phoenix late in the summer of 2019, rock formations, patches of forest, and serene spaces dotting the landscape. Xan and I were enjoying one of our cherished drives together. Laughter and conversation flowed freely as we navigated the scenic route, immersing ourselves in the natural beauty surrounding us.

Our chats moved effortlessly from movies to in-depth analyses of television shows and scripts. Xanny, with his keen eye for artistic detail, reveled in breaking down narratives, dissecting them piece by piece. This particular day we found ourselves engrossed in a discussion about *Game of Thrones*.

"I can't wait to start streaming the next season, dad!" Xanny exclaimed with a broad grin and sparkling eyes. "It's such a crazy moment the way a zombie ice dragon destroyed a thousand-year-old wall in like minutes! Just like 'Boom!' and it's gone! Thousands of years, just gone, like that!" Xan snapped his fingers with a flourishing motion.

"Yes, son, it's going to be pretty great," I replied. "We just gotta make sure we watch it together somehow!"

As we drove on, my thoughts shifted from ice dragons to the chill of Xan's bipolar diagnosis just a few months earlier. His restlessness had become more noticeable during our TV time. Pacing back and forth, he would resist our invitations to sit, insisting "No, I'm fine," while continuing to pace as we watched.

I seized the moment to check in on his emotional well-being. Taking advantage of a curve around a particularly large rock formation, I asked directly, "Xanny, how have you been feeling lately?"

Still grinning from our *Game of Thrones* discussion, he paused, and the sparkle in his eyes softened.

"I've been okay, Dad," he began, his voice carrying a weight I couldn't quite place. "Just figuring things out, you know? School's a bit tough sometimes, but I'll be fine."

His grin reappeared, a mask he wore well. "Just the usual stuff, dad. School, life, future plans. You know, the works."

But "the works" seemed heavier than he let on, and I couldn't shake the contrast between the vibrant young man engrossed in TV fantasy worlds and the subtle unrest he just admitted.

"You know what I mean, Xan," I said. "How have you been feeling? How's the medication been working? I've been worried because I've read up on it, and it says that sometimes it can make . . . ," I paused, "it can sometimes cause suicidal ideations."

Xan bristled at the statement.

"I just want to make sure you're okay. You know how much you mean to all of us."

"It's okay, Dad. You don't have to worry about me. I got a plan," he said surprisingly firm, his eyes filled with determination.

"Really?" I smiled questioningly.

"Yeah, Dad, this is all about putting in the work. I'm going to work out, get my blood flowing, get rid of these extra pounds, and, plus, I'm going to start eating clean. Diet has so much to do with all this. Don't worry, dad. I got a plan."

He stared off, his brow knitted. "I just don't want you both to worry. You and Mom have given me so much. I love you guys so much, and I don't want to burden you."

His words pricked my heart. "You're never a burden to me, Xan. You're one of the best things in my life. Just know I'm here for you. Anything you need, Xanny, I'm here for you. Just say the word, and I'll drop everything and come running."

I smiled. "Even if I have to run straight or in zigzags, I'll be there!"

Xanny laughed at the reference to a *Game of Thrones* character who ran in a straight line instead of zigzagging to avoid being hit by an arrow.

"I still can't believe it, and I'm not over it yet either, Dad! That's all he had to do—just zigzag!"

Our laughter filled the air, dissipating the tension as we navigated another curve in the drive, making our way home. The stress and worry also dissipated in the joy of simply being together with my son.

***

THE ABYSS OF DESPAIR

The next thing I knew, I was on the ground, huddled in a corner, my body wracked with sobs that felt like they were tearing me apart. These were not mere tears; they were the deep, profound wails of a soul laid bare, a father's heart shattered into a million pieces.

How could this be? The reality was too much to bear. Our son, our beloved Xanny, was gone, and with him, a part of us that we would never regain. At that moment, time ceased to exist. There was only the crushing weight of loss, a void so profound that it threatened to consume everything in its path. The chaos and yelling and screams faded behind me, receding like a distant storm.

"It finally happened," I kept repeating to myself, the words pulsing through me like a relentless heartbeat. The very thing I had feared the most, the unspeakable event that had lurked in the shadows of my thoughts, had come to pass. The fear that had whispered in quiet moments, in the still of the night, had become a deafening reality.

My beloved boy had taken his own life.

In that corner I realized that my mind and heart had been in a constant battle against a truth that my soul had already known. Deep down, in a place where fear and love intertwine, I had always sensed the fragility of Xan's existence, the precarious balance of his life on a tightrope of hope and despair.

A torrent of emotions overwhelmed me—grief, disbelief, guilt. Thoughts zig-zagged through my mind, memories of Xanny flashing in rapid succession, his laughter, his dreams, his struggles. Then, the diagnosis—the therapy sessions, the medication. A journey we embarked on together but now one from which he would never return. I sobbed even harder with the gnawing, relentless guilt of a father who wondered if he could have done more.

In my mind, I replayed our last conversations, our final moments together, searching for signs I might have missed. The weight of regret was suffocating, a heavy cloak that threatened to crush me under its burden. Could I have been more present, more attentive? The questions haunted me, each one a sharp jab at my already fragile state.

People around me tried to offer comfort, their words trying to bridge the gap of my sorrow. But their voices seemed distant, their touch, a faint sensation against the overwhelming tide of my grief. I had a profound sense of isolation. It was as if I had been transported to a parallel universe where everything looked the same but was fundamentally altered. I had never felt so alone. I was adrift in an ocean of loss, unable to see the shore, unsure if I even wanted to.

In this moment of absolute devastation, in this new dimension, time no longer existed. The past, present, and future merged into a singular point of pain. The pain was not just emotional; it was physical. My heart literally ached with the ebb and flow of each sob. My body felt heavy, every movement an enormous effort. Grief had manifested in every part of me, consuming me whole as it dragged me, helpless, into a cruel new reality.

It was in this abyss of despair that I realized the depth of my love for my son. A love so profound, so integral to my being, that it transcended his physical presence. He was not just my son; he was a part of my soul, an indelible mark on the fabric of my existence, a connection now deeply severed.

The loss of a child is not something one recovers from; it's something you endure, day by day, moment by moment. In that enduring, there is no room for anything but the stark, raw reality of your shattered world.

In that corner there was no thought of moving forward, no consideration of healing. Those were concepts too distant, too alien in the face of such profound loss. All that existed was the moment, the excruciating pain of now, the devastating reality of a future without Xanny, my son.

There was only grief.

Chapter 3:

MY LIFE IN TWO HALVES

———

The Suicide Bridge

On a radiant spring day, the car filled with the light chatter of my children, Xan and Ava, as we approached the Coronado Bridge. The sun cast a brilliant sheen over the water, the bridge arching majestically into the sky, a testament to the beauty that San Diego mornings often hold. But as we ascended the roadway, a shadow of my past flashed through my mind, briefly taking me back to a darker time in my youth.

Heading into my early twenties, my world was steeped in turmoil. Isolated from a community I once called mine, estranged from my family, and grappling with depression, I faced the abyss of despair. Back then, driving up this bridge represented not a passageway but a potential endpoint, a place where the weight of my existence teetered on the edge as I contemplated a tragic leap.

Yet today, surrounded by the laughter and presence of my children, the bridge transformed from a symbol of despair to one of continuity and hope. I am washed over with gratitude for the journey from those desolate thoughts to these moments of familial joy, grateful for the strength that pulled me back from the brink so I could enjoy this drive with Xan and Ava and the potential of our shared day together.

Suddenly, though, the car ahead of us came to an abrupt stop at the bridge's highest point. What followed was unimaginable and surreal. In one swift motion, the driver flung open her door, sprinted to the ledge, and disappeared over the side. Our collective gasp filled the car in a moment of shared disbelief.

Once the immediate chaos settled, security personnel directed us forward. As we drove off the bridgeway in silence, I glanced at Xan and Ava and asked if they needed to talk. Their quiet assurances did little to dispel the sense of shock that enveloped us all.

As we continued driving, Coronado greeted us with its usual splendor, seemingly oblivious to the tragedy that had just unfolded. The pristine beaches, elegant palms, and serene ocean vistas painted a portrait of tranquility, a stark contrast to the horror we had just witnessed.

The dissonance between our peaceful surroundings and the woman's desperate act was jarring. As we moved through the scenic routes of the island, the beauty around me felt almost surreal, starkly contrasting with the turmoil that had unfolded on the bridge. I grappled with how someone could feel so trapped in darkness. This led me to a somber realization: One can be in the midst of the most beautiful surroundings and still feel utterly isolated in their own personal prison of despair.

Note: The Coronado Bridge, known for its picturesque views connecting San Diego to Coronado Island, holds a somber distinction. It is recognized as the second most active site for suicides in California, following the Golden Gate Bridge. This stark reality contrasts sharply with the bridge's scenic beauty and serves as a poignant reminder of the hidden struggles that many individuals face.

***

UNCHARTED TERRITORY

October 27, 2019, stands as a stark demarcation in my life's narrative, dividing it into two distinct eras: the time before and the time after Xanny's passing. My life, up to that fateful day, was a tapestry of varied experiences—adversity, despair, growth, joy, and a deepening connection with those around me. I had weathered storms, celebrated victories, and believed I understood the spectrum of life's challenges.

However, the loss of my son plunged me into uncharted territory. The adversity I faced in the wake of this tragedy was unlike anything I had encountered. It was an ordeal that reshaped my understanding of suffering and resilience. Reflecting on my life before this loss provides context to the transformation that ensued. The joys and struggles of my earlier years, once defining aspects of my identity, took on new meanings in the aftermath of Xanny's death.

By sharing the contours of my life before this defining moment, I hope to illustrate how profoundly my world was altered. The lessons and strengths I had accumulated were tested in ways I never anticipated. This isn't just a story of loss but also a narrative about how a life, rich with its own unique trials and triumphs, can be irrevocably changed by a single, devastating event.

My intention is to offer insight into how the fabric of a person's existence can be rewoven in the aftermath of profound tragedy.

THE EARLY YEARS

Born into the warm embrace of a Mexican family in Southern California, my life began in a blend of cultures—a rich Mexican heritage and the quintessential American dream. My parents, Ignacio Leon III and Eunice Escamilla Leon, were committed to raising us in faith and family, the very best way they knew how.

Despite our roots, Spanish was a language heard but not spoken in our household. This peculiarity set us apart in a community where Spanish was common. It was particularly noticeable in the tiny church where my father served as an assistant pastor. The church, a modest gathering of about thirty people, conducted its services entirely in Spanish. Imagine the irony—three kids, part of a predominantly Spanish-speaking congregation, yet not fluent in the language themselves. We attended church four times a week, each service lasting three hours, and twice on Sundays. Since the age of nine, I played keyboards during each service. It was a rigorous routine, but it fostered in me a deep sense of faith and community.

My father, a man of unwavering faith and integrity, always carried a bright smile and joyous nature that could lighten the heaviest of hearts. His positivity was infectious, a trait that helped our family navigate the many challenges we faced.

My mother was the backbone of our home life. Her days were spent in a whirlwind of activity, tending to me and to my two brothers, Nathaniel and Michael, and later to our little sister Debbie. Her hands were always full and at times overwhelmed; but her love, dedication, and self-sacrifice for all of us was never in question.

I was actually born in Augsburg, Germany, where my father was stationed at the time of my birth. He had joined the army straight out of high school, marrying my mother shortly before he started his enlistment. Life in the military suited him well until, sadly, he lost four of his fingers while working on a diesel engine. The accident led to an honorable discharge and our subsequent move back to Southern California.

Despite what must have been a profoundly dark period for him, grappling with the loss of his fingers, he never let his struggles cast a shadow over our family life. It was remarkable; my father emerged not just intact but seemingly unscathed in spirit. He didn't allow his injury to be a crutch or an excuse for anything less than living life to the fullest. It was as if by sheer will and faith in God that he refused to let his difference define him or diminish his role as a father and husband. He was, in every essence, a whole person exuding an aura of completeness that defied his physical condition. I was extraordinarily proud of his strength and character.

His sense of humor, in particular, was a testament to his unbreakable spirit. He would often quip with a chuckle, "I can't give you a high five, but how about a thumbs-up instead?" And he was always ready when someone asked him to give them a hand, responding, "Hey man, I'm a little short-handed myself!"

It was a joyful, gentle reminder that life, despite its trials, could still be approached with a smile and a positive outlook.

The foundation laid during those early years was filled with joy and contentment. My days were rich with the simple pleasures of youth—riding bikes until the sunset painted the sky, playing soccer on weekends with my dad as the encouraging coach, and enjoying the warmth of family meals. We were well cared for, with a stable home that was grounded by God and family. This period of my life, with its unique experiences and victories, defined my upbringing. It was much like Xanny's own cheerful and carefree early years. Yet, as I transitioned into my mid-teens, I felt a palpable shift.

TEENAGE TURMOIL

When I was fourteen, our family moved to Moreno Valley. It was the early 1990s, and my father had decided to establish a new church of his own there. As the church began to take shape, so too, did my role within it. Transitioning from a young member of the congregation to its primary keyboardist placed me at the heart of our worship services, further intertwining my passion for music with my family's spiritual mission. However, this new chapter also brought with it the challenges of adolescence and the looming shadow of my father's legacy, setting the stage for a complex journey through my high school years.

Entering high school, I was acutely aware of the chasm between the expectations set by my father's legacy and my own sense of self. My dad, with his high school history as an acclaimed athlete, his commanding presence, and his unwavering faith, stood as a towering figure in my life. He was not only revered in our family for his spiritual leadership but also remembered fondly by those who knew him for his athletic prowess and charismatic personality. In contrast, I found myself wrestling with feelings of inadequacy on multiple fronts.

Physically, I was noticeably shorter than him, a difference that felt like a glaring reminder of the ways in which I didn't measure up. Spiritually, while I was deeply involved in our church, playing the keyboard and contributing to our services, I couldn't shake the feeling that my faith and my persona lacked the depth and conviction that characterized my father's.

This internal narrative that I wasn't enough—neither the athlete nor the man of faith he exemplified—was compounded by a belief that my value in our family, particularly in my father's eyes, was predominantly tied to my musical contributions to the church. It felt as though my worth was measured by what I could do rather than who I was. This perception, though misguided in hindsight, was a reality I lived with, feeding into bouts of depression that I kept hidden from those around me. Very few people, if any, were aware of the struggles I faced. It's a poignant reminder of how personal battles can be so deeply concealed that even those close to us remain oblivious—a parallel to what later unfolded in Xanny's life.

At the time, these thoughts were deeply ingrained beliefs that shaped my self-image and my interactions with the world. The discrepancy between who I was and who I thought I needed to be to gain my father's full approval and pride led me down a path of silent suffering. It was a struggle masked by the facade of the dutiful son and talented keyboardist, hiding the turmoil that lay beneath.

Looking back, I can see the misconceptions that clouded my

judgment. My father's love and pride in me were not as conditional as I believed. However, during those formative high school years, this belief was a heavy burden, coloring my experiences and pushing me into a solitude marked by depression. The journey through this time was a complex interplay of striving for acceptance, grappling with personal identity, and the pursuit of self-worth beyond the shadows of perceived expectations.

This facade of normalcy shattered when I was sixteen. A family disagreement spiraled out of control, and in a moment of rebellion and desperation, I dropped out of high school and ran away to San Diego, where my grandparents and my mother's side of the family lived. It was a rash decision, driven by a maelstrom of emotions and a yearning for escape. This act of defiance marked a significant turning point in my life. It hastened the emancipation that often accompanies a young man's departure from home, particularly under strained circumstances, setting me on a path filled with lessons, hardships, and the reality of facing the world on my own.

While in time all was forgiven and bridges were eventually rebuilt with my parents, the path to reconciliation took time. It wasn't the ideal way to forge independence, and it certainly did nothing to alleviate the mental health struggles I was already facing.

A FAMILY OF MY OWN

Not too many years later, at the tender age of eighteen, I found myself standing at the altar with Debra Esperiqueta, my amazing, talented, and beautiful wife. The story of how I came to marry my wife unfolds like a narrative steeped in serendipity and underscored by the transformative power of love.

To describe Debra is to speak of radiance and resilience. Her personality shines brightly, her demeanor defined by an undeniable strength and unshakeable fortitude. Her musical talent, especially her remarkable voice, complemented her vibrant character, making her not just a presence to be reckoned with but a force of nature in her own right.

Our paths crossed in the most unlikely of venues. I had taken on the role of helping to form and lead the choir at the new church I was serving, unaware that Debra was set to do the same. It's never simple when two leaders, each with distinct views and approaches, strive to guide the same ship; so our initial interactions were fraught with confrontation and arguments as we each endeavored to steer the choir according to our own vision. These disputes, though fiery, masked an underlying current of mutual respect and admiration for each other's passion and dedication to music.

What began as a professional rivalry slowly transformed into something much deeper, a connection that neither of us could have anticipated. Our many disagreements served as the backdrop against which our feelings for each other gradually took root and flourished. It was as if we were the unwitting stars of our own romantic comedy, complete with tension, laughter, and, ultimately, love. The process through which we fell in love was emblematic of the very nature of love itself: unpredictable, challenging, and profoundly beautiful.

Debra and I discovered that our confrontations were not clashes of ego but collisions of passion. As we navigated through our differences, we learned to appreciate the depth of each other's commitment to music and ministry. This mutual respect became the foundation upon which our relationship was built. Our shared love for music, once a battleground, turned into a symphony of harmonious understanding and affection.

Marrying Debra was a testament to the idea that love can emerge from the most unexpected circumstances. It demonstrated that even through moments of disagreement and challenge, there exists the potential for a deeper connection, one that is strengthened rather than weakened by adversity. Debra became not just my partner in music but in life. Our journey together, from leading choir rehearsals to leading a life shared in love, serves as a reminder that sometimes, it's the most challenging beginnings that lead to the most beautiful endings.

CLIMBING THE CORPORATE LADDER

Marriage ushered in a new set of responsibilities. The pressure to provide was immediate and intense, steering me towards a career in the mortgage industry. I started as a real estate agent, then a loan officer, navigating the complexities of real estate and finance, driven by the need to build a stable life for my young family. It was during this time not long after our marriage that we welcomed our son, Alexander, into the world, a joyous event that only fueled my determination to succeed.

Alexander's arrival was like a burst of light, infusing our lives with an indescribable joy and a profound sense of purpose. His first breath was not just the beginning of his life but also the dawn of a new chapter for Debra and me. Every smile, every innocent gaze from those bright eyes reaffirmed the depth of our love and the responsibility we now shared.

The birth of our son also deepened my resolve to provide and to succeed, not just for myself but for this precious life we had brought into the world. His presence in our lives was a constant reminder of the beauty and fragility of life, motivating me to strive for greatness in every endeavor. He was more than just our child; he was a living embodiment of our love, a symbol of hope and the future, as was our beautiful daughter, Ava, born a few short years later.

It wasn't just about financial stability anymore; it was about excelling, pushing boundaries, and redefining my capabilities. I decided to pursue a bachelor's degree in 2015 and a master's degree in 2017, which qualified me for even higher positions. My career trajectory took a significant upward turn as I continued to advance into leadership roles. Leadership changed everything. It taught me the power of influence, the importance of vision, and the impact of effective decision-making.

Alongside my professional ascent, I dove headfirst into the world of self-help and positive thinking, recognizing their potential to fundamentally reshape my approach to life's challenges. Influential figures like Les Brown and Tony Robbins became beacons of transformation, guiding me through a profound process of personal development. Their insights into changing one's thinking to change one's life struck a chord with me, leading to a deliberate and purposeful application of their teachings.

The allure of self-help and positive thinking stemmed from a deep-seated desire to evolve beyond the constraints of my past experiences and current mindset. Brown's stories of triumph over adversity and Robbins' methodologies for achieving personal excellence provided more than inspiration; they offered practical tools and strategies for mental and emotional overhaul. By adopting their philosophies, I initiated a significant shift within myself, moving from a place of self-doubt and limitation to one of empowerment and possibility.

This transformation was a fundamental change in how I perceived and interacted with the world around me. I began to dismantle the mental barriers that had confined me, adopting a new inner narrative that championed my strengths and potential. Positive thinking and self-help principles taught me that no matter how difficult your past, it doesn't have to determine your future. I learned to view challenges as opportunities, to envision success vividly, and to practice gratitude for the journey, thus fostering a mindset of growth and abundance.

The impact of this shift was evident in every facet of my life, particularly in my career, where promotions and recognition became tangible manifestations of my internal growth. These achievements were direct outcomes of my commitment to applying the principles of positive thinking and self-help, illustrating the profound effect of mindset on reality.

I felt I had achieved the pinnacle of my career when I took on a high-level management position for a multinational financial services company. Overseeing two locations and more than 225 employees, I felt like I had conquered the world. Life was more than just prosperous; it was a dream realized: a beautiful family, a successful career, and a future that seemed limitless.

But life, as I had come to understand, was unpredictable.

The sudden, tragic day that tore my son from our lives was like being thrown into an unknown arena, forced to face challenges I had never imagined. Everything I had built, every belief I had held, was put to the ultimate test. This moment marked the end of the first half of what had seemed like a picture-perfect life and the beginning of an uncharted one filled with chaos, uncertainty, and unfathomable grief.

Chapter 4:

FALLOUT FROM THE UNFATHOMABLE REALITY

The Arena

In the comfort of my home, life was a warm embrace. Surrounded by the laughter of my family and the familiar sights and sounds of everyday contentment, I basked in what felt like a never-ending atmosphere of peace and love. The days were a tapestry of simple joys and shared moments, a picture-perfect tableau of happiness.

But then, without warning, it all changed.

One moment I was wrapped in the security of my cozy existence, and the next, I found myself somewhere else entirely—a place foreign, cold, and uninviting. Disoriented, I struggled to make sense of my surroundings. The gentle hum of my home was replaced by an ominous silence, broken only by distant, echoing chants. I was no longer in the sanctuary of familiarity; I had been abruptly uprooted, abducted from my life, and thrown into the shadowy darkness of an unknown world.

As my eyes adjusted to the dim light, a stark, new reality began to set in. I stood in an arena, vast and dark, with dust swirling around my feet, each particle a silent witness to my confusion and fear. The gate before me, a monolithic structure, creaked open slowly, revealing the unknown that awaited me.

A chilling sense of dread washed over me. The air grew thick with a palpable sense of evil. From the depths of this foreboding abyss emerged creatures, the likes of which defied all realms of my understanding. They were grotesque parodies of life, twisted and misshapen, cloaked in shadows that seemed to writhe and squirm with a life of their own. Their eyes glowed with a malevolent fire, burning with an intensity that spoke of hunger, of a relentless desire to consume and destroy.

The creatures advanced, their movements discordant and jarring, as if they were not bound by the laws of nature that govern our world. The ground seemed to shudder with their every step, a morbid drumbeat to the chaos that was unfurling. I realized these were not just monsters; they were manifestations of my deepest fears, my darkest thoughts, brought to life in this hellish landscape.

I could feel the panic rising within me, a primal, all-consuming terror that clenched at my heart. My breaths came in short, sharp gasps, each one a battle as the air itself felt thick and hostile. As the creatures encircled me, their presence suffocating and overwhelming, I understood with crushing clarity that this was my new reality.

In the back of my mind, a voice screamed for a way out of this nightmare. But as I scanned my surroundings, a horrific realization dawned on me—there was no escape. The arena was a closed circle, a trap from which there was no exit. The walls, once my hope for refuge, now stood as silent sentinels, witnesses to the impending doom that approached. The comfort and warmth of my past life were gone, replaced by this arena of despair and confrontation. Here, in this place where hope seemed a distant dream, I was to face the very essence of my fears. This was not just a battle for survival; it was a struggle for my very soul, a test of my will to endure and overcome the darkest depths of despair.

***

ALTERED STATES

In the immediate aftermath of the devastating news, a surreal haze enveloped my world. The contours of reality blurred, as if I were viewing life through a frosted glass. The shock of losing my son gripped me with an icy hand, paralyzing both thought and emotion.

In those early days of grief, the world felt unreal, and I, a ghost within it, untethered and adrift. The shock was a buffer against the full force of my loss, but it was also a barrier, keeping me from beginning the true process of mourning. In this blurry reality, I stood at the precipice of a journey through grief, a journey that promised no easy passage but was necessary for the healing that I could not yet envision.

Time became a nebulous concept, with minutes stretching into hours, yet passing in what felt like mere seconds. The normalcy of life around me seemed grotesquely disjointed, a stark contrast to the turmoil raging within.

I remember wandering through those first few days after Alexander's death in a daze, actions and decisions made on autopilot. The physical world around me existed in a dimension of its own, the people in it living a regular existence, happy, or at least undisturbed—a painful reminder of the normality that had been so cruelly snatched from my grasp. The chasm between me and the rest of the world seemed to widen with each passing moment, deepening my sense of isolation and disbelief.

As I grappled with the raw shock, my mind, in its attempt to shield me from the full impact of my loss, had altered my sense of reality, leaving me in an altered state of consciousness that was both a defense mechanism and a curse. Moments of lucidity were interspersed with stretches of numbness, each phase bringing its own brand of pain. The clarity was piercing, a sharp reminder of my loss, while the numbness was a hollow respite, offering temporary oblivion but no true escape.

THE WEIGHT OF WORDS

When the time came to communicate the tragic news, each word felt like a physical burden, heavy with the gravity of what had happened. Making those phone calls to family and friends was an ordeal that drained me of what little strength I had mustered. With each call, I had to relive the reality of my son's passing, each repetition a hammer blow to my already fragile state of being.

The act of informing others was not just about sharing the news; it was an act of making the unimaginable real. As I spoke the words, "We've lost him," it was as if I was hearing them for the first time myself. The finality those words carried was overwhelming, each syllable a stark reminder of the permanence of our loss.

After the personal phone calls, I decided to post about my son's passing on social media.

"Friends, We have no easy way to share. Today we lost our first born, our son, Alexander. He was the heart of Debra and I, as well as Ava. Xan battled depression for a long time. At this point I have more questions than answers. Our hearts ache for one more hug, one more text, one more call. Our faith is in Him, the one who created us. Energy does not dissipate, it only transfers. Xanny went from this world to the next. Baptized six years ago today. We will see you again my sweet, sweet boy. I know this in my heart."

Ignacio Escamilla Leon is with **Debra E-Leon**
October 27, 2019 · ⚙

Friends, We have no easy way to share. Today we lost our first born, oldest son, Alexander Leon. He was the heart of Debra Lion and I, as well as Ava. Xan battled depression for a long time. At this point I have more questions than answers. Our hearts ache for one more hug, one more text, one more call. Our faith is in Him, the one who created us. Energy does not dissipate, it only transfers. Xanny went from this world to the next. Baptized 6 yrs ago today. We will see you again my my sweet sweet boy. I know this In my heart.(our last photo).

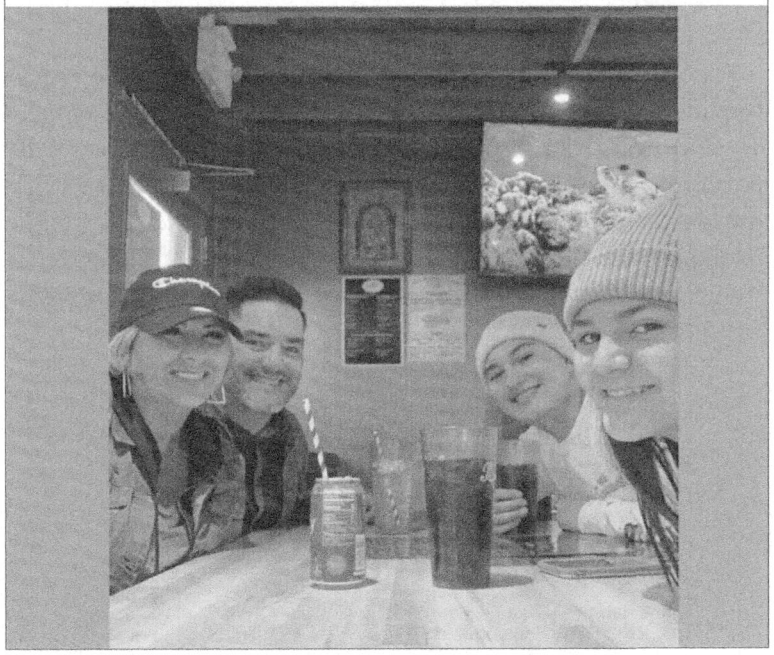

Typing out the message felt like sending a distress signal into the vastness of space, a call for acknowledgment, for shared grief in a world that felt increasingly distant.

The reactions from family and friends came like a deluge, each phone call and message a testament to the impact my son had on those around him. The shock, heartache, and grief in their voices mirrored my own in an outpouring of shared sorrow.

It was during these conversations that the waves of grief hit me the hardest. With each tearful recount of my son's impact on their lives, the reality of his absence was hammered home. The grief I felt was not mine alone; it was a collective mourning, a community brought together by loss, and with it, a semblance of solace.

Knowing that my son's life had touched so many others provided a small comfort in the midst of overwhelming sadness. These conversations, though heart-wrenching, were a necessary part of the grieving process, a way to begin coming to terms with the loss as a family, as a community. They were the first steps in a long journey of healing, one that we would walk together, each step marked by our love and memories of a life taken too soon.

Chapter 5:

COPING WITH REALITY

The Shadow of Absence

Christmas time was here, our first without our Xanny.

As I stepped out of my car, the chilly embrace of the winter air wrapped around me, a stark contrast to the warmth I once felt during this festive season. The parking lot was dimly lit, shadows playing across the asphalt, mirroring the darkness that had settled in my heart. Each step towards the store felt heavier than the last, a physical manifestation of the dread that weighed down my soul.

The bright lights of the store felt jarring as I walked through the automatic doors. Christmas decorations adorned every corner, festive music played over the speakers, and shelves overflowed with holiday cheer. This should have been a time of joy, of preparation for family gatherings and celebration. Instead, each ornament, each strand of tinsel, was a painful reminder of the void that now existed in my life.

I moved mechanically through the aisles, picking out decorations and food, trying to adhere to some semblance of normalcy. But the act of preparing for Christmas without my son was a torture I hadn't anticipated. The looming dread of celebrating without him, of facing the empty space where he should have been, was overwhelming.

As I passed the toy section, a haunting reminder stopped me in my tracks. There among the shelves of games and gadgets was the video game section.

Xanny loved his video games. I was instantly transported back to the Christmas when I gave him a Nintendo. I saw myself holding a controller with him, playing and laughing, flashes of his excited face raining through my mind and heart.

The breakdown came without warning. Tears blurred my vision as I stumbled to the back of the store, seeking refuge in a quiet corner. The walls closed in around me, and the festive music turned into a distant echo. I was alone with my grief, uncontrollable sobs racking my body.

In that solitary space, hidden away from the world, I wept uncontrollably. It was a moment of raw vulnerability, a moment where the facade of strength I had been trying to maintain crumbled entirely. The memory of my son, so vivid and painful, was a reminder of all that had been lost. There, in the back of that store, I grappled with the reality of my first Christmas without him, a season that once held so much joy now shadowed by his absence.

***

THE STRUGGLE FOR SANITY

As the reality of my son's absence continued to cement itself in my life, I found myself in an ongoing struggle to maintain a grasp on sanity. The world around me seemed to move on, but I was stuck, mired in a state of grief that threatened to consume me whole. The pain was unrelenting, a constant companion that shadowed my every moment.

There were times when the line between grief and madness blurred, when the sorrow was so deep and engulfing that it felt as if I would lose myself to it entirely. My mind oscillated between moments of acute clarity, where the loss felt unbearably real, and stretches of numbing disconnection, where everything seemed distant and surreal.

Long after the funeral, when social conventions dictated a return to normalcy, my grief remained as raw and pervasive as ever. Tears would come unexpectedly, often triggered by the smallest reminders—a photo, a familiar scent, a snippet of a song. These moments of sudden sorrow were like cracks in the dam, brief but intense reminders of the depth of my loss.

Denial, too, was a frequent visitor in my journey of grief. Despite the undeniable reality that Xanny was no longer with us, part of me kept hoping for a miracle, for some twist of fate that would reverse the irrevocable. This denial was not born out of ignorance but out of a desperate desire to escape the pain, to find respite in a fantasy where my son was still alive and well.

THE FINALITY OF ABSENCE

As the immediate shock began to wane, I was faced with the daunting task of grappling with the permanence of my son's absence. This realization crept in slowly, a gradual and painful awakening to the countless moments and experiences that we would never share again. Each day brought its own set of reminders: the empty chair at the dinner table, the silence of a room once filled with laughter, the future plans that would remain unfulfilled.

In the solitude of my grief, memories of the past began to emerge with a haunting clarity, each one tinted with the pain of newfound understanding. These recollections, once sources of joy and warmth, now cast long shadows over my heart. They were no longer mere reminiscences; they had become reflections of a life irrevocably altered.

I would find myself lost in thoughts, revisiting moments and conversations with my son, each tinged with the regret of hindsight. The laughter we shared, the milestones we celebrated, the everyday exchanges—all were now infused with a bittersweet poignancy. These memories were a testament to the bond we shared, yet they also underscored the enormity of the void his absence had created.

I found myself mourning not just for the person my son was but for all the things he would never be. The weight of each uncelebrated birthday, each unattended milestone, pressed down on me. Simple joys, such as watching a show we used to enjoy together or planning to attend a baseball game, became sources of profound sorrow. These activities, once taken for granted, now stood as stark reminders of his absence.

This period was characterized by a series of "never agains." Never again to hear his voice. Never again to share a joke. Never again to offer advice or encouragement. Each "never again" was a poignant echo of loss, reverberating through the emptiness left behind. The realization of these permanent absences was a harsh confrontation with reality, a reality where his presence was irrevocably missing.

The cumulative effect of these realizations was overwhelming. Each day seemed to bring a new layer of understanding of what his absence truly meant. It was as if I was slowly peeling back the layers of a wound, each one revealing a deeper, more painful truth, each opening up new depths of sorrow.

In facing these truths, I began to understand that grieving was not a linear process but a complex journey through various stages of realization and acceptance. Mourning each lost future moment was not only an act of grief but also an act of love, a recognition of the deep bond that would always exist between my son and I, despite his physical absence. This period of realization was a crucial step in my journey through grief, a painful yet necessary path towards coming to terms with a life forever changed.

Chapter 6:

ENEMIES AT THE GATE

The Belt Incident

"Do you need anything?" Debra asked Xanny as she prepared to go shopping one day.

"Just a belt. Mine broke," he replied nonchalantly.

Thinking it a bit odd, Debra asked, "How did it break?"

Xanny shrugged as high school teens often do. "I dunno, I just broke it."

Dismissing it at the time, what seemed then a minor inconvenience now loomed over us with a sinister significance. Xan had used a belt to commit suicide in his dorm room. Could the belt he broke then been an early, failed attempt at taking his own life?

This chilling revelation cast a dark shadow over me. It raised a tormenting question: Had there been signs of his inner turmoil that I had missed? This insight into a past incident, once overlooked, now became a focal point of my grief, a painful reminder of the complexities and nuances of Xan's internal struggles. How long had he been suffering? How many failed attempts had he made before finally succeeding? Had God intervened to save him before? Why hadn't He stopped him that last time?

Both harrowing and enlightening, the broken belt incident forced me to confront the reality that there were aspects of my son's life that I may not have fully understood. In the aftermath of his death, this left me searching for clues on my journey of self-discovery and reflection which became an integral part of my grieving process, a way to connect with my son's memory and come to terms with the many facets of our shared life and his untimely departure.

***

RETURNING TO THE PRESENT REALITY

One of the most daunting aspects of my new reality was the uncertainty about the future. "What do I do next?" became a recurring question, echoing in the silence left by my son's absence. This question was not just about daily routines or long-term plans; it was a deeper inquiry into the meaning and purpose of my life in the wake of such a monumental loss.

Each day as I faced this question, I felt a profound sense of aimlessness and despair. The path I had been on, the future I had envisioned, was no longer relevant. I had to find a new direction, a new reason to move forward, but the way was shrouded in grief and uncertainty. Coping with this new reality was more than just a challenge; it was an existential journey, a search for a way to live in a world that had been forever changed.

At this point in my journey, the wounds of my loss were still raw, the pain as fresh as if the tragedy of Xan's suicide had occurred only moments ago. The dust of my shattered world had yet to settle, but amid the lingering fog of grief, certain adversaries began to emerge with stark clarity. These "enemies at the gate," once obscured by the initial shock and chaos of loss, were now revealing themselves, each impacting my life in profound and challenging ways.

Pain: An Ever-Present Shadow

Pain was the most constant of these enemies, a relentless shadow that followed me every moment. It wasn't just an emotional ache but a physical presence, a tightness in my chest that reminded me of what I had lost. This pain was a constant echo of my son's absence, a relentless reminder that life would never be the same.

Hopelessness: A Glimpse Into A Bleak Future

Hopelessness had begun to creep in, casting a long, dark shadow over my thoughts of the future. Where once there were aspirations and dreams, now there was a void. The future, which should have been filled with possibilities, now seemed barren, stripped of the joy and purpose my son had brought to my life.

Guilt And Negative Self-Voice: The Inner Critic

Guilt, accompanied by a chorus of negative self-talk, was a formidable enemy. It whispered accusations and fostered doubts about my actions and decisions. This inner critic constantly questioned whether I could have done something different, something more, to alter the tragic course of events. The possibility that Xanny's struggles might have been hidden in plain sight was a heavy burden, laden with guilt and "what ifs."

Anger: A Burning Flame Within

Anger smoldered within me, sometimes burning bright and fierce. It was an anger directed at the world, at fate, and even at myself. This rage was a tempest, sometimes simmering just below the surface, other times erupting in moments of overwhelming emotion.

Bargaining: The Fruitless Negotiation

I found myself bargaining with reality, caught in a cycle of "what ifs" and "if onlys." This futile negotiation with the past was an attempt to find an alternate reality where my son was still alive, a desperate wish to turn back the hands of time.

Detachment From Reality: The Allure Of Numbness

Detachment presented a seductive escape from the pain. It tempted me to disengage, to retreat into a shell where the harshness of reality could not reach. This numbness was a double-edged sword, offering temporary relief but at the cost of disconnecting from the life that continued around me.

Destructive Nihilism: The Abyss Of Despair

In my lowest moments, destructive nihilism whispered that nothing mattered anymore. The belief that no future could be bright without my son threatened to unravel the very fabric of my being, undermining any sense of purpose or hope.

As these enemies became more apparent, their impact on my life more pronounced, I understood that facing them was not just necessary but crucial for my survival. This battle with my inner demons was as important as any physical challenge I had ever faced. It marked a critical point in my journey: overcoming these adversaries was the key to finding a path through my grief towards a semblance of peace.

UNDERSTANDING THE ENEMIES WITHIN

As I grappled with each of these formidable enemies, a moment of introspection allowed me to step back and analyze what I was truly experiencing. This wasn't just about enduring grief; it was about understanding the multifaceted nature of my suffering. Each of these emotions—pain, hopelessness, guilt, anger, bargaining, detachment, and nihilism—represented a different aspect of my struggle, a different facet of my journey.

I began to see these emotions not just as obstacles to overcome, but as integral parts of my healing process. They were the enemies at my gate, yes, but also guides in disguise, each one highlighting a crucial area of my inner self that needed attention and care. Recognizing their presence was the first step in learning how to navigate through them.

Acknowledging the existence of these emotions was painful. It required me to confront truths about myself and my situation that I would have rather left unexplored. However, it was also an act of empowerment. By naming these feelings, by understanding their roots and their impact on my life, I was taking back some control over my grief.

I realized that if I didn't actively confront and push back against these emotional adversaries, they had the potential to consume me completely. This wasn't going to be an easy battle. Each enemy required a different strategy, a different approach. But the mere act of preparing for each confrontation was, in itself, a form of healing.

Understanding the enemies within marked a turning point where I moved from passively enduring grief to actively engaging with it. I understood now that this battle was crucial for my survival. It was about more than just finding a way to live with my loss; it was about finding a way to emerge from it with a new understanding of myself and the world around me.

As I moved forward, I carried with me the knowledge that this journey was not just about battling grief but about transforming it. The road ahead was still uncertain and undoubtedly filled with challenges, but I was no longer walking it blindly. I was armed with the awareness of what lay ahead and the determination to face it head-on.

A CALL TO THE READER

In sharing this chapter of my journey, I extend a hand to you, friend, who might be navigating your own path through grief. If my story resonates with you, know that you are not alone in this struggle. The enemies at the gate—pain, hopelessness, guilt, anger, bargaining, detachment, and nihilism—are universal adversaries in the journey of loss. But from my experience, here's how you can use them as allies in your healing process.

Recognizing What's At Stake

It's crucial to recognize what's at stake in your own battle with grief. The emotions and challenges you face are not just obstacles to be overcome; they are integral to your healing process. Understanding them is the first step toward reclaiming control over your journey through sorrow.

The Importance Of Acknowledging And Confronting

Acknowledge each emotion, understand its roots, and confront its impact on your life. This process of acknowledgment and confrontation is a powerful tool in your arsenal against grief. It's a step toward healing, a step toward a future where your loss is a part of you but does not define you.

Empowerment In Your Journey

As you move forward, remember that this journey is as much about transformation as it is about healing. You have the power to emerge from your grief with a deeper understanding of yourself and the world. The road ahead may be fraught with challenges, but armed with awareness and determination, you can navigate it with a newfound strength.

A Pivotal Moment For Change

Battling the enemies at the gate is a pivotal point in your journey. It's where you transition from merely enduring grief to actively engaging with it. Embrace this challenge, for it is crucial for your survival and growth. It's about finding a way to live with your loss and finding a way to let that journey transform you.

In closing this chapter, I urge you to consider what lies ahead for you. The battles may be daunting, but they are also opportunities for growth and understanding. You have the strength to face them, to push back against the darkness, and to find your way through. Your journey, like mine, is unique, but the destination is the same—a place of peace, of understanding, and of renewed strength.

Chapter 7:
A CRISIS OF FAITH

A Moment of Profound Doubt

The kitchen was filled with the mundane noises of daily life—the humming of the refrigerator, the ticking of the clock—as I gathered my coat and car keys. Planning a quick run to the store, I called out to Debra, "Need anything else besides milk?"

She stood by the window, her gaze lost somewhere in our backyard, her mind seemingly miles away. "Babe, are you there?" I asked, a hint of concern creeping into my voice as I noticed her distant demeanor.

There was a long pause. The air felt heavy, charged with unspoken thoughts. Then, without turning from the window, her voice came, almost a whisper, yet piercing through the quiet of the room.

"What if it's all a lie? What if none of it's real?"

I froze, the keys now insignificant in my hand.

"We've given our whole lives to Jesus," she continued, her voice beginning to tremble. "We must have sung a thousand songs, given thousands of dollars, and all of it for what?"

Her words hung in the air, heavy with despair.

I approached her slowly, but before I could reach her, she turned to me, her eyes brimming with tears.

"If it's not real, then we'll never see Xan again."

As she broke down, I wrapped my arms around her, trying to offer comfort. Yet, within me, her words reflected a spark of doubt that had been attempting to take hold of me privately, a silent, creeping uncertainty that echoed her fears:

What if it was all a lie?

***

QUESTIONING BELIEFS UNDER DURESS

The cool wind against my face did little to ease the turmoil within as I rode my motorcycle down the road Xanny and I used to travel together. It was our road, a place where we shared thoughts, dreams, and laughter. Now, it was just me, accompanied by a deafening silence and a heart heavy with grief.

As the familiar landscape blurred past me, a surge of anger welled up inside. It was a raw, burning emotion that demanded acknowledgment. In that moment, speeding down the road we once shared, I realized the true focus of my anger: it was directed at God.

This wasn't just a fleeting emotion; it was a deep-seated fury born from a sense of betrayal. I had always been a man of faith, believing in a just and loving God. But now, in the wake of my son's passing, that belief was shrouded in doubt and anger. How could a benevolent God allow such a tragedy? Where was the divine intervention I had prayed for?

The more I dwelled on these thoughts, the more the anger grew, fueled by unanswerable questions and the stark unfairness of my situation. I had dedicated my life to serving God, to being a good man, a good father. Yet, here I was, riding alone, engulfed in a pain that seemed to mock my devotion.

The road stretched out before me, but it offered no escape from the turmoil inside. With each mile, the reality of my crisis of faith became clearer. This was no ordinary doubt; it was a fundamental questioning of everything I had believed in. It was a confrontation with a God who I felt had abandoned me in my hour of greatest need.

As I rode on, the anger simmered within me, a tempest that threatened to consume my faith. This ride was not just a physical journey; it was a journey into the depths of my soul, a journey that would challenge the very foundations of my belief.

As the road unfolded before me, my mind raced back to the times when I had witnessed God's intervention in the lives of others. I remembered how He had pulled my teenage brother out of a dangerous gang lifestyle, an answer to the fervent prayers of my parents. Their faith had been a beacon, guiding him back to safety. I had seen firsthand the power of prayer, the miracles that seemed to follow those who waited on and trusted in God.

Yet, as I reflected on these moments, a bitter realization took hold of me. I had been praying for Xan for months before he passed, anointing him with prayer oil each morning every chance I got, believing with all my heart that God would protect him, that He would guide him through his struggles. My faith had been absolute. It never crossed my mind that God might let me down.

But He had. The pain of that realization was like a physical wound. I felt betrayed, not just by the loss of my son but by the silence of a God I had so devoutly served. How could a loving God ignore the prayers of a father pleading for his son's life? The question gnawed at me.

My thoughts took a darker turn, wandering into the territory of divine judgment. Was this tragedy a punishment from God? Had I somehow failed in my service to Him? Did I neglect God and His calling, and was this punishment for not pursuing him deeper? These thoughts built a wall around my heart, a barrier of fear and doubt that separated me from the very One that had always been my source of strength and comfort.

The anger I felt was intertwined with this fear, creating a tumultuous storm within me. God had always been my refuge, my guide through times of trouble. But now, He felt distant, unreachable beyond the wall of anger and fear in my heart. This disconnect left me adrift, unmoored from the spiritual anchor that had always held me steady.

Riding along that road, the memories and doubts swirling in my mind, I realized that my crisis of faith was not just about questioning God's actions. It was about confronting the foundations of my belief, the very essence of my relationship with Him. This was a journey through the valley of shadows, a journey that would bring me face to face with questions that threatened to unravel the fabric of my faith.

Reckoning With Anger And Worship

In the aftermath of my son's passing, as the initial shock gradually faded, I found myself in a complex emotional landscape where deep-seated anger coexisted with a commitment to worship. This duality was confusing and often painful. How could I continue to worship a God I was so angry with? How could I sing praises and offer prayers to a deity who, in my eyes, had failed me in my most desperate hour?

My anger towards God was not a fleeting emotion; it was a persistent, gnawing presence that colored my days and nights. Yet, despite this anger, I couldn't abandon my practice of worship. The rituals and prayers were ingrained in me, a part of who I was at my core. But now, these acts of devotion were tinged with a sense of bitterness and confusion.

This period of reckoning was one of the most challenging phases of my crisis of faith. I struggled to reconcile my feelings of betrayal with my desire to maintain a connection with God. The anger I felt was a barrier, yet my worship was a bridge—albeit a fragile one—that I hoped could somehow keep me connected to the God I had known my whole life.

CONFRONTING THE UNTHINKABLE

The worst of these thoughts, the one that haunted me relentlessly, was the notion that all my anger, all my faith, might be futile because God didn't exist. This thought was alien, almost blasphemous to someone who had spent a lifetime steeped in faith. I had been a leader, a youth pastor, a musician in the church since I was nine. My life had been a testament to God's presence—leading others to Him, praying for the lost and the hurting. God had been as real to me as the air I breathed.

Yet now, faced with the silence following my son's passing, this thought gained a foothold in my mind: What if the reason God hadn't answered my prayers for Xan was that He wasn't there at all?

This was a terrifying possibility. It shook the very foundations of my existence.

As Debra had pointed out, if God didn't exist, the implications were twofold—and devastating. Not only had we dedicated our lives to what might be a fable, but it also meant we would never see Xan again. He would not be in a better place, not in heaven or with the angels but lost forever in the void, a memory fading into the darkness.

The weight of this thought was crushing. To entertain the possibility that my son's laughter, his energy, his essence could just cease to exist was unbearable. It was a notion that threatened to consume me with despair, a black hole that threatened to swallow not just my faith but my very will to find meaning in life.

This was the abyss I found myself staring into, a precipice that beckoned with a cold, unyielding truth. The journey of faith I had walked so confidently until now suddenly seemed like a path shrouded in mist, leading to an unknown, perhaps non-existent destination.

But in the depths of this despair, a small, defiant part of me resisted. I couldn't accept this conclusion without a fight, without seeking, without questioning. This was not just a crisis of faith; it was a crisis of existence, of meaning, and of purpose. I had to find answers, not just for my sake, but for the memory of my son, for the life we had built around a belief that had suddenly turned fragile.

I needed answers. Answers to questions I never dared ask before. This hunger, this desperate need, became the driving force in my darkest hours. And it was during this search for answers that I began to notice them—the seeds of hope. They had been there all along, subtly planted, waiting for the right moment to reveal themselves. These seeds, I realized, were not just random occurrences; they were signposts, guiding me back to a path I thought I had lost—and grounding me for the journey ahead.

THE PATH TO RECONNECTION

The journey back to Xan's dorm to gather his belongings was one I had been dreading. The thought of returning to the place where he had lived, laughed, and dreamed was almost unbearable. But it was there, amidst the heaviness of my heart, that the first seeds of hope were unexpectedly sown.

As I stepped onto the floor of his dorm, something I can only describe as a gust of wind rushed past me, almost as if clearing the path ahead. In that breeze, I felt more than just a physical chill; a whisper reached deep into my soul. The words were clear and resonant:

"I allowed him to come home because I love him."

The message was powerful, profound, bringing with it a moment of inexplicable relief. For the rest of that day the dread that had weighed on me lifted, replaced by a sense of peace that defied understanding. It was a comfort I could only attribute to the still small voice of God.

This was just the beginning. A couple of days after Xan's passing as we prayed for a sign that he was okay, something extraordinary happened. As we uttered his name, the fire alarms throughout the house inexplicably went off. It was as if the universe itself was responding, acknowledging our plea in the most unforeseen way. This was the second seed, a moment that defied natural explanation, yet offered a glimmer of hope amidst our despair.

The third seed was planted at the funeral home. It was the last time I would lay my physical eyes on Xanny. He lay there, peaceful, as if merely asleep. In that moment, instead of being overwhelmed by grief, an unexpected serenity enveloped me. It was a deep, internal assurance that Xan was okay, that we would see him again, and be reunited. This feeling, in stark contrast to the sorrow of the occasion, was a profound reassurance planted firmly in my heart.

In the midst of all the turmoil, I hadn't realized that God was planting these seeds of hope for me. They were like breadcrumbs scattered along the path of my grief, guiding me, offering me glimpses of light in the darkest of times. Each of these experiences, though they made little sense in the natural world, were beacons leading me back, helping me to find my way home. It was a profound realization: in our moments of deepest despair, there are always seeds of hope, and God, in His mysterious ways, helps us to find them.

Seeking Solace in Scripture

As I embarked on this journey of rediscovery and reconnection, my first refuge was in the scriptures, the sacred texts that had been a part of my life since childhood. These verses and passages, once familiar and comforting, now demanded a deeper examination. I was no longer just reading; I was seeking, dissecting every word for a hidden meaning, a message that might have eluded me before.

One Scripture that stood out during this time was from the New Living Translation version of 1 Corinthians 15:5, a passage I had read countless times but now saw in a new light: "Our bodies are buried in brokenness, but they will be raised in glory. They are buried in weakness, but they will be raised in strength."

This verse, in its starkness and promise, struck a chord within me. It spoke of transformation, of a journey from mortality to something greater, something divine.

This was more than just a comforting thought. It was a profound insight into the nature of our existence—the idea that our physical end was not the ultimate conclusion. In the context of my grief, this scripture offered a glimmer of hope, a possibility that Xan's journey was not over, but transformed into a different existence beyond my understanding.

I dove deeper, exploring other passages, seeking out connections and meanings. Each scripture became a piece of a larger puzzle, a step towards understanding the bigger picture of life, death, and the divine. This process was not just about finding comfort; it was about building a foundation of understanding, a framework within which I could begin to reconcile my grief with my faith.

As I immersed myself in these sacred texts, I felt as if I was engaging in a dialogue with the divine. Each verse, each line, was a part of a conversation that spanned the ages, offering wisdom, solace, and at times, challenging my preconceived notions. It was a journey back to the very essence of my faith, a rediscovery of beliefs that had been shaken, but not shattered, by my son's passing.

Seeking Shared Experiences

In my search for understanding and solace, I also turned to the stories and experiences of others that resonated with my struggle. Among the most impactful were those of Rick Warren and his wife, Kay, whose journey through grief, especially after the loss of their son, mirrored my own in many ways.

An author, pastor and founder of Saddleback Church, an evangelical Baptist church in Lake Forest, California. Rick's insights and Kay's strength and wisdom became a source of guidance and comfort. I dove into their teachings, their interviews and their writings, seeking anything that could shed light on my path. Their openness about their struggles, doubts, and ultimately, their steadfast faith amidst unimaginable pain provided a template for my own healing process.

It was not just their words that provided comfort, but the realization that others had walked this path before me and had somehow found a way to navigate through their grief. In their stories, I found echoes of my own pain and glimpses of a possible future where the overwhelming grief could be transformed into something bearable, even meaningful.

This part of my search was more than just a quest for knowledge; it was a lifeline, a way to feel connected to a community of souls who had suffered similar losses. It was a reminder that while each journey through grief is unique, the threads of pain, doubt, and eventual healing are common to all.

Understanding Life Beyond the Physical Realm

This led me next to the exploration of near-death experiences (NDEs), seeking further understanding of life beyond the physical realm. I watched dozens, maybe hundreds, of accounts from those who had found themselves on the brink of death. Each story was a window into the profound mysteries of existence and, possibly, the afterlife.

These NDEs, while unique in detail, shared common traits that resonated deeply with me. Many described feelings of intense peace, well-being, and love, experiences of leaving their bodies and observing themselves from an outside perspective. There were accounts of moving through darkness towards an indescribable light, encountering deceased loved ones, and even having life reviews.

What struck me most was the sense of unconditional love and acceptance that seemed to envelop those who had a near-death experience. This aspect, in particular, brought comfort, suggesting that Xan might have been embraced by such love. The idea that he might have experienced such peace and beauty in his final moments gave me an indescribable sense of solace.

Equally fascinating were the reports of enhanced mental clarity and the sensation of being drawn into a tunnel or darkness, only to emerge into a realm of light and knowledge. These experiences challenged my understanding of life and death, urging me to consider the possibility of consciousness existing beyond the physical body.

These accounts, though varied, painted a picture of an existence much larger and more complex than our earthly understanding. They offered a glimpse into a world where the soul's journey did not end with physical death but transformed into a new state of being.

As I delved deeper into these stories, my own grief began to intertwine with a newfound sense of curiosity and wonder about the mysteries of life and death. The more I learned, the more I began to see these NDEs as potential guideposts on my own journey of understanding and healing.

Moments of Spiritual Confirmation

In the midst of my quest for understanding, I began to encounter a series of events and seemingly serendipitous moments. Each one seemed to appear just when I needed it most, much like manna, the bread-like substance that fell from Heaven and fed the Israelites. These occurrences, both small and profound, came to me during prayer, reflection, and everyday life, each serving as a bridge over the chasms of doubt and despair.

There were numerous instances that defied simple explanations or dismissals as mere coincidences. Some were subtle, almost whisper-like experiences that left me with a sense of peace or a fleeting moment of clarity. Others were so stark and astonishing that they could not be attributed to chance alone.

There was a time when I was running and caught a glimmer of a shiny quarter on the ground. The year on it was 1999, the year Xan was born. And once as we were leaving for a family trip that he would have been on with us, the song "1999" by Prince came on the radio. At other times we found feathers in the car or saw license plates with "Xan" on them.

I felt a deep conviction that these were signs from God, perhaps even messages from Xan, telling us, "I'm okay. I'm on the other side. I'm so happy here, and you will be too one day. I see you, please don't cry." With each passing moment and each new sign, the burning ember of my dwindling faith was slowly, steadily rekindled.

Whether simple coincidences or divine interventions, these moments of what some would call "spiritual confirmation" played a crucial role in reshaping my faith. They were reminders that, even in our darkest hours, we are not alone. Internally we seek signs, but that does not mean someone or something isn't seeking us out to be found. There is a presence, a love, that holds us, guides us, and speaks to us in ways that are often beyond our comprehension.

It was during this time that my understanding of faith began to evolve. I found myself moving away from the rigid structures and doctrines that had previously defined my beliefs. Instead, I was drawn towards a faith rooted in the unconditional love of God for His children—a love that transcended our human understanding, our mistakes, and our imperfections. Each experience, each moment and confirmation, served to strengthen my resolve to keep seeking, keep praying, and keep believing in the vast, unfathomable love of a God who was, in His own mysterious ways, leading me back home.

The Wayne Dyer Moment

My ongoing search for answers eventually led me to the works and words of various self-help experts and motivational speakers, among them Dr. Wayne W. Dyer, author of the groundbreaking book, *The Power of Intention*. I had been studying it and following Dr. Dyer for several months. I also had resumed and found respite in my daily runs, which allowed me a space for reflection and contemplation, and it was while running one day I had what I like to refer to as my "Wayne Dyer Moment."

As I ran that day, I listened to him explain a scientific discovery. Researchers probing the origins of existence within an atom found that our DNA appears to emerge from what seems like nothingness at an infinitesimally small scale. Understanding this as a scientific truth given the blueprint of our DNA, Dyer continued that while it may appear we emerged from "nothingness," in fact, we come from something he referred to as an unseen "source."

This concept deeply resonated with me, revealing a profound intersection of science and spirituality. It echoed the teachings I had always embraced: We don't just materialize out of a void; we originate from a source far greater than what our physical senses can perceive.

As I contemplated what I was hearing, my pace slowed from a run to a walk and then to a complete stop. In that moment, a realization took root in my heart with undeniable clarity. This idea transcends the materialistic view of life's origins, hinting at a cosmic interplay between the physical and the metaphysical, the known and the unknowable. It suggests that the emergence of life from this "nothingness" is not an accident but a glimpse into a grand, orchestrated design, possibly overseen by a Creator. This concept reshapes not only our understanding of where life comes from but also the very essence of our existence, pointing to a divine intelligence that maps out life's journey long before it unfolds in the tangible world.

This was the spiritual truth that connected the dots between science and faith for me. It was a moment where science and spirituality didn't just coexist; they converged, affirming my belief in a Creator who is both the author of the physical laws of the universe and the spiritual truths that govern our existence. It was an affirmation that my search for answers, my wrestling with faith amidst grief, was not in vain.

My "Wayne Dyer Moment" was more than an intellectual epiphany; it was a spiritual awakening. The realization that we came from somewhere, from Someone, bridged the gap I had felt between my faith and the physical realities of our existence. In this moment of clarity, I felt a renewed connection to God, a renewed understanding of my faith. It was a turning point in my journey of healing, a beacon of light guiding me back to a path of reconciliation with my beliefs and with my God.

It was my concrete affirmation of the existence of a Creator, a Master Designer behind the tapestry of life. This newfound understanding brought with it a reassurance that life, and indeed Xan's life, was part of a grand, divine design. Even more so, if we literally came from our Creator with physical DNA, plans for expression and life, and even spiritual plans for purpose, it was easy to believe we would return to Him when we left this tangible world. I could once again stand upon what I had already known—that there is a life after this one that I can't see with these mortal eyes.

And when I finally arrived there, Xanny would be waiting for me.

This wasn't just a hopeful notion; it was an unshakeable conviction that brought with it an indescribable peace. The doubts and turmoil that had clouded my faith for so long were dispelled in an instant. It was as if a longstanding question that had haunted my heart was finally answered, not with words, but with a deep, inner knowing.

This understanding resonated with the biblical truth expressed by the Apostle Paul in 2 Corinthians 4:18: The things we see are temporary, but the things we do not see are eternal.

The pieces of my spiritual puzzle, which I had turned over in my mind for months, now fell into place with a satisfying click. The realization that our existence is part of a larger, more mysterious tapestry, where the physical and the spiritual intertwine, dawned on me not just as a concept, but as a living truth.

As I stood in that moment of awakening, a profound sense of resolution washed over me. The struggles with faith and the piercing pain of loss were still part of my journey, but they were now underpinned by an unyielding bedrock of belief. This was more than acceptance; it was a transformation, a transition from grappling with belief to resting in the certainty of God's eternal promise.

This was not merely the end of a chapter but a significant milestone on a continuing journey. It provided a foundation for healing, a solid ground from which to view the trials and tribulations of life. Like a weary traveler who finally finds their way after a long journey, I felt an overwhelming sense of relief and gratitude. It was the beginning of a renewed faith, deeply anchored in the assurance of God's unconditional love and the eternal nature of our souls.

Back On Track

This moment marked a turning point, a shift from uncertainty to a peaceful certainty in my faith. It was a testament to the power of enduring belief and the profound peace that comes with truly settling one's heart in the hands of God.

In this newfound understanding, a powerful symbol emerged in my life—the image of a train track. This symbol became a representation of my path towards healing and reconnection. Just as a train track stretches towards a destination, often unseen in the distance, so, too, did my journey stretch towards a reunion with my son and a deeper understanding of the divine.

This train track, with its singular, determined direction

symbolized the journey to our heavenly Father, with whom I believed Xan now resided. It was a visual reminder that despite the twists, turns, and sometimes obscured view, there was a destination—a place of peace, reunion, and eternal love. Changing all my screensavers to this image, I was constantly reminded of this path and the hopeful destination it promised.

The Thread of Healing

As I traveled along this track, I discovered that the process of healing was akin to pulling on a thread in a complex tapestry. With each pull, hidden patterns and designs began to emerge. Each unraveling thread, once found, became a template for my healing, revealing insights and truths that were previously obscured by my grief and pain.

This template was not just about finding answers to my questions but about understanding the greater design of life, love, and existence. It was about seeing the interconnectedness of all things, recognizing that our physical lives are just one part of a much larger, spiritual journey. Each day, each experience, each serendipitous moment added to this tapestry, creating a pattern that guided me towards a deeper understanding of God's unconditional love for His children.

As I continued to pull on this thread, I realized that the journey was not about reaching a final destination but about the journey itself. It was about the process of healing, growing, and understanding. The train track, the symbols, the moments of living confirmation were all leading me towards a place of peace, acceptance—and a renewed connection with God.

Chapter 8:

PUSHING BACK

Climbing Mountains

As Debra and I trekked up the mountain, the cool breeze was a stark contrast to the warmth we once felt on such hikes. It had been only a month since we lost Xanny, and our hearts were still heavy with grief. Each step felt like a reminder of the void left in our lives.

Reaching a clearing, a sound, all too familiar, pierced the calm—the sound of weeping. Instinctively, we moved towards it, driven by a shared understanding of that profound sorrow. There, we found a woman, sitting alone, her cries echoing the pain that had become our constant companion.

"Are you okay?" we asked, our concern genuine as Debra gently placed a hand on her shoulder. The woman looked up through tear-stained eyes. "My son," she gasped between sobs. "My son . . . he's gone forever."

A silent understanding passed between Debra and me. We knew that pain, that irrevocable loss. As the woman's tears subsided, leaning into Debra's embrace for comfort, we dared to ask, "How long has it been?"

Her next words struck me like a physical blow, "Eight years."

I stepped back. Eight years? The thought reverberated through my mind. The intensity of her grief was as raw as if the loss had just occurred only days before. How could one endure such pain for so long?

Debra's compassion never wavered as she continued, "Do you have other children?"

"Yes, four," the woman whispered.

Another jolt to my heart. For eight years, this woman had been trapped in her sorrow, her other children relegated to the periphery of her grief. The thought of enduring such unending agony, of possibly inflicting such prolonged pain on my own family, was unbearable.

As Debra consoled her, I tried to process what this meant for us, for our future. The encounter was a stark warning—a glimpse into a future where, if grief remained unchecked, pain could morph into something all-consuming. This couldn't be our fate. There had to be a way to master this grief, to prevent it from becoming a relentless tormentor.

The mountainside encounter was a crossroads, a moment of clarity amidst our own suffering. It underscored the urgency of finding a path through our pain, not just for our sake but for those who still needed us. The mountains, which had always symbolized strength and resilience, now bore witness to our resolve to seek a way forward, to tame the all-consuming grief that threatened to define our existence.

***

THE NEED FOR CHANGE

As the days turned into weeks and months, the relentless grip of grief began to manifest in more than just emotional pain; it started to take a toll on my physical health. I could see the signs—my body deteriorating, the sleepless nights, pain in unusual places—all pointing to a body and mind under siege. The realization that my grief was not just an emotional battle but a physical one too was both startling and sobering.

If I were to survive, to somehow navigate through this tempest of sorrow, I needed to make a change. I couldn't continue on this path of self-neglect; it was unsustainable, a road that led only to further despair.

The necessity to be present and supportive for my family became a powerful motivator to change. My family, also grappling with grief, needed me. I needed to be there for them, to be a pillar of strength even if I felt anything but strong. I had to find a way to push back, to re-engage with life, not just for my sake, but for theirs.

My Daughter, Ava

In the wake of our profound loss, the encounter with the grieving woman on the mountain left an indelible mark on my psyche. It served as a stark reminder of the potential long-term impact of unaddressed grief, not just on oneself but on those who remain a part of our lives. This realization brought into sharp focus the need to heal, not just for my own sake, but for the sake of my family, especially my daughter, Ava.

In her early middle school years, Ava was at a crucial juncture in life, a time when the presence and guidance of a father were indispensable. The idea of her navigating these formative years with only a shell of her father, haunted by grief and loss, was unbearable. The thought of her growing up with the shadow of not just her brother's loss but also her father's absence, was a wake-up call.

It became increasingly clear that surrendering to despair would not only dishonor the memory of my son but would also rob Ava of a father who was fully engaged in her life, one who could share in her joys, guide her through her struggles, and be a steady source of love and strength. The realization that she needed me, coupled with the understanding that I needed her just as much, was a powerful motivator in my journey towards healing.

Ava's youthful innocence, her resilience in the face of our family tragedy, and her need for a stable, loving father were the catalysts that drove me to seek a path to wholeness. She became a symbol of the future, a beacon of hope, reminding me that life still held beauty, potential, and reasons to keep moving forward. The responsibility to be there for her, to guide her, and to watch her grow into the remarkable person she was destined to be was a compelling force that spurred me to find the strength to rise each day, to face my demons, and to slowly rebuild myself.

Ava, with her youthful wisdom and love, taught me a valuable lesson: that even in the darkest of times, there are reasons to heal, to grow, and to embrace life again. She was, and continues to be, a reminder that love in its purest form that can guide us back to light, to hope, and to a renewed sense of purpose.

My Wife, Debra

I am forever grateful to Debra, my extraordinary partner, for showing me through her actions that it is possible to respond to grief with love, purpose, and a relentless pursuit of life. Her strength and resilience have been my inspiration, teaching me that even in the face of the greatest loss, we can choose to live with intention and hope. She is not just my wife; she is the living embodiment of the power of love to heal, to inspire, and to change the world.

Debra's approach to grief was a stark contrast to mine. A beacon of strength, compassion, and unyielding love, her response to our devastating loss was nothing short of extraordinary, a testament to the depth of her character and the boundless capacity of her heart.

While I grappled with the urge to retreat into the shadows, to hide from reminders of our son, she chose a path illuminated by his memory. She saw his pictures not as symbols of pain but as celebrations of his life, vibrant echoes of his presence that deserved to be seen and to be remembered. Her ability to find joy in his memory, to keep his spirit alive through photographs and stories, was a profound act of love and courage.

Debra's response to our son's passing was a revelation to me. It was a reminder that even in the depths of despair, there is a choice in how we respond to the world around us. She chose to open her heart, to embrace the pain and transform it into something meaningful, something beautiful. She chose to let the world witness the joy our son brought to us, the beauty he added to our lives, and the change he could still inspire by starting the Xan You Matter Foundation, a beacon of hope for young individuals battling depression and suicidal thoughts, helping sons and daughters so families don't lose another one. Her resilience transformed our shared pain into a mission, channeling her grief into a cause that would honor our son's memory and potentially save lives—including, very likely, mine.

Watching Debra navigate her grief with such purpose and passion was a turning point for me. Her dedication to honoring our son's life, her commitment to our family, and her unwavering passion for helping others became my guiding lights, urging and pulling me out of my own darkness. She took on the role of founder and president of Xan You Matter, and I serve as vice president. In the beginning, supporting and helping her was very hard, a constant, painful reminder of what happened to Xan. But her example showed me that there was another way to deal with our loss, a way that didn't involve succumbing to despair but rather embracing life and honoring our son's memory through positive action.

Returning to Work

The prospect of returning to work also emerged as a key factor in my healing journey. My job had always been more than just a means to an end; it was a part of my identity, a realm where I had felt competent and confident. Work had given me a sense of purpose, and I realized that reclaiming this part of my life was crucial for my healing journey. The thought of returning to a routine, to a world that had remained static while mine had collapsed, was daunting. Yet, I knew it was necessary. It was a stepping stone to finding some semblance of normalcy, a pathway back to a life that wasn't defined solely by grief.

Returning to work was not just about resuming professional duties; it was about reclaiming a part of my identity that had been overshadowed by grief. It was an opportunity to engage with a world that, though unchanged in my absence, offered a different kind of challenge—one that I felt equipped to handle. The thought of immersing myself in work was a beacon of hope, a chance to momentarily step away from the shadows cast by the enemies at the gate.

On my first day back, the familiar surroundings of the office brought a strange sense of comfort mixed with disquiet. As I walked through the corridors, greeted by the nods and sympathetic smiles of my colleagues, I felt a pang of alienation. Each interaction was a reminder of the life I once led, uncomplicated by the immense loss I now carried with me.

To manage the complexities of grief in a professional setting, I developed strategies that allowed me to honor my emotions while fulfilling my responsibilities. This included setting aside time for reflection, openly communicating my needs with my team, and allowing myself moments of vulnerability. These strategies weren't just coping mechanisms; they were integral to maintaining a sense of integrity in my role. They helped me to build a bridge between the person I was before the tragedy and the person I had become—a leader shaped by loss but not defined by it.

DESIRE TO FULFILL DESTINY

The pain of losing Xan was unrelenting, but I started to see a glimmer of a different kind of purpose, an understanding that his life and what he meant to me could be a catalyst for something meaningful. Despite the fact that my entire world had stopped spinning, ever so slowly the cogs had begun to turn again. My people, my purpose, were emerging from the faintest of shadows. I knew they were the reasons I needed to keep pushing back to continue on my journey to healing.

I began to see that Xan's passing, though unbearably painful, need not be in vain. There was a chance here to transform this profound loss into a force for something positive, a way to honor his memory in the actions and choices I made moving forward.

This was about finding a way to make his absence matter and fulfilling his destiny, to ensure that the love and lessons he imparted continued to resonate in the world, through me. So, I started an organization of my own—Make Shift Happen. This organization is dedicated to utilizing the tools I've detailed in this book to help those trapped in trauma. Our goal is to help them move beyond just surviving their grief and despair, to a place where they can heal, succeed, and thrive once again.

The idea of turning my son's passing into a purposeful catalyst was a delicate one, filled with complex emotions. It wasn't a solution to the grief but a way to navigate through it. It offered a means to counter the creeping sense of nihilism, the feeling that nothing mattered anymore. In honoring Xan's memory, in allowing his influence to continue through my actions, I could find a way to keep a part of him alive. It provided a direction at a time when I felt most lost, a reason to push through the pain, and a way to ensure that Xan's legacy continued in this world.

This phase of my life, challenging as it was, helped me to emerge more aware, more empathetic, both as an individual and a professional. It underscored the undeniable truth that our personal experiences, especially those marked by loss, can shape us in profound ways.

Chapter 9:

THERAPIES FOR HEALING, PART I

Battling Despair

A s the first rays of dawn crept through the blinds, casting a thin, quiet light across my room, my preparedness was a silent rebellion against the pain that awaited me. For weeks, my body had succumbed to a state of paralysis, a physical manifestation of the emotional turmoil within. However, this day was different. I had laid out my running clothes the night before, a small but significant step towards breaking free from the chains of grief.

As the memories began their daily assault, I resisted the urge to surrender to tears. Instead, I found myself moving almost mechanically, slipping into my sweatpants and exercise shirt, and stepping out into the cool, early morning air. My body, still aching from the inactivity of the past weeks, protested with every step, but I pushed forward.

Xanny . . .

The act of running was initially a mechanical motion, a forced effort to escape the paralysis that gripped me. But as I picked up the pace, the floodgates of emotion burst open. Tears streamed down my face, not from despair this time but as a release. As I ran faster, driven by a surge of anger and frustration, each stride became a battle, a fight against the overwhelming sense of loss that had been my constant companion.

With every sprint, I felt a rush of emotions—anger, sorrow, defiance—propelling me forward. My breaths grew labored, my calves ached, and my chest burned with the exertion. Yet, amidst this physical struggle, there was a moment of clarity, a fleeting instant where the pain in my heart was momentarily forgotten. It was in these strides, between the physical discomfort and the struggle for breath, that I found an unexpected respite.

As I slowed to a stop, panting and drenched in sweat, I was enveloped by a sensation unfamiliar in recent times—a sense of accomplishment. Along with the soreness and exhaustion, there was a glimmer of hope, however faint. For the first time since my son's passing, I had battled the paralysis, the hopelessness, and emerged victorious, even if just for the duration of that run.

This run marked a breakthrough—a realization that I could fight against the stagnation that grief had imposed upon me. It was a revelation that, in the act of physical movement, in the battle against my own body's resistance, I could find brief moments of escape from the emotional pain. This small victory was the first step towards a larger battle against the despair that had consumed me.

***

Author's Note: The following insights and suggested therapies for healing are rooted in personal experience and research into coping mechanisms for grief and emotional distress. While I draw upon general knowledge, I have not cited specific scientific sources, as my focus is on sharing relatable experiences and practical guidance for readers navigating similar challenges. The concepts discussed are grounded in recognized findings and have been adapted to reflect my own journey and understanding.

PHYSICAL ACTIVITY AS A PATHWAY TO HEALING

As the weeks turned into months after my son's passing, it felt as though I had been relentlessly battling in the arena with no respite in sight. My days were consumed by managing the pain as best I could, yet it seemed like I was merely existing, not living. The reality was, much of what had been happening was happening to me, and I was barely keeping afloat in the turbulent waves of grief and hopelessness.

But there came a turning point, a moment of stark realization: I needed to do something, anything, to break free from the unyielding grip of my sorrow. The pain, though inescapable, sparked a desperate need within me to find some semblance of control, to seek out a lifeline within all the chaos.

It was in this desperate state that led me to the healing power of sweat, the first therapy I embraced to find my way out of the darkness.

The Power of Sweat

The experience of that morning's run was a profound revelation in my journey through grief. It was more than just physical exertion; it was a crucial step in my emotional healing.

The role of physical exercise in managing emotional pain cannot be overstated. Engaging in regular physical activity, be it a brisk walk, a jog, or a session at the gym, serves as a natural antidote to the heavy cloak of sorrow. The act of moving your body, of pushing through physical limits, mirrors the mental and emotional resilience needed to face life's challenges. It's about channeling the pain into something constructive, transforming it into a source of strength.

Incorporating Exercise into the Healing Process: The Benefits of Physical Exercise

Incorporating regular physical activity into your daily routine can be a vital component in the healing process. It doesn't have to be intense or prolonged; even moderate exercise like walking or yoga can be immensely beneficial. The key is consistency and finding an activity that resonates with you.

Exercise became my ally in the battle against grief. It provided moments of escape, opportunities for emotional processing, and a pathway to rebuilding my physical and mental strength. For anyone navigating the turbulent waters of loss, I recommend considering physical activity as a valuable tool in your healing arsenal. It's not a complete solution, but it's a powerful component of a holistic approach to recovery and well-being, offering many benefits:

1. **Stress Reduction through Endorphin Release:** Engaging in physical activity prompts our bodies to release endorphins—natural chemicals that help improve mood and reduce stress. For those grappling with grief, this biochemical reaction can be a vital tool, offering a natural form of relief in emotionally tumultuous times.

2. **Enhanced Emotional Processing:** There's something profoundly therapeutic about physical exercise. It demands our full attention, yet amidst the physical exertion, our minds find clarity. Personally, I've often experienced significant insights during a challenging run—moments when my mind and heart seem to spontaneously piece together unresolved emotions.

3. **Channeling Anger and Frustration:** Intense physical activities, like hitting a punching bag, offer more than just physical benefits. They provide a safe and productive way to express and manage difficult

emotions, such as anger and frustration. Reflecting on my own experiences, I recall how running faster when frustrated not only helped manage my emotions but also gave me a way to confront an otherwise intangible adversary.

4. **Improving Sleep and Physical Well-Being:** Regular exercise contributes significantly to improved sleep quality—a crucial aspect for anyone, but especially vital during times of grief. Establishing a consistent routine not only helps alleviate sleep disturbances but also enhances overall physical health, making it easier to face each new day.

5. **Neurochemical Changes and Brain Health:** Physical activity isn't just about improving our present state; it also promotes the growth of new neurons, a process known as neurogenesis. This brain development is associated with improved cognitive functions and emotional regulation, helping us maintain mental clarity and emotional stability during challenging times.

6. **Building Resilience and Confidence:** Each physical challenge we overcome through exercise doesn't just strengthen our bodies—it builds our emotional resilience. Overcoming these challenges fosters a sense of achievement and self-confidence, crucial for navigating the complexities of grief. Like leveling up in a journey of personal growth, every small victory counts.

THE POWER OF A VISION STATEMENT

In the wake of profound loss, the future I once envisioned shattered into countless pieces. The passing of my son not only took a part of my heart but also fractured the very framework of my expectations for the days ahead. In this new reality, where grief loomed large, the future became an obscure landscape, clouded by a pervasive sense of hopelessness and despair. Every once-cherished dream seemed to dissolve in the wake of my tragedy, leaving me in a void where even the simplest joys lost their luster.

In those early months of navigating my grief, I found myself caught in an endless loop of loss and fading hope. Desperate for a lifeline, I scoured books and videos, seeking anything that offered a new way to view the remainder of my life. This search led me to a challenge that would become a turning point: the creation of a personal vision statement. It was a daunting task, one that required me to confront the reality of my existence within this altered landscape and to dare to believe in a future still worth living.

The journey to craft this vision was riddled with internal conflict. Part of me feared that by looking forward and constructing a new vision, I was somehow leaving my son behind, relegating him to the past. This internal battle raged for weeks, leaving me stranded in a no man's land between a paralyzing grief and the inability to move forward.

Then, one seemingly typical morning, something within me shifted. I had a breakthrough, suddenly understanding that I couldn't remain anchored in that painful spot any longer.

Embracing this newfound resolve, I allowed myself the freedom to dream once again. In my heart, I held onto the belief that my pain had a purpose, that there was still a plan for my life. I recognized that the depth of my suffering could be the very catalyst for a renewed destiny. With pen in hand, I began to outline everything that still resonated within me—aspirations for my wife, my daughter, my community, and beyond.

As I crafted my vision statement, it evolved into more than a mere collection of goals and dreams; it became a profound inquiry into the core of my being. Questions like "Why am I here?" and "What truly matters to me?" led me to the essence of my existence, to the heart of my purpose. This process was a journey to the center of my soul, unearthing truths that had been overshadowed by my loss.

Reading my vision statement became a daily ritual, a mantra that guided my mornings and evenings. Over time, this practice began to shift my mental outlook. The vision I had penned down started to paint a new picture of what was possible, offering a glimpse of hope amidst the fluctuating tides of grief. The vision became a compass, guiding me back to a sense of self, to a life where hope flickered in the distance, beckoning me forward.

Crafting Your Personal Vision Statement: A Pathway Through Grief

The creation of a personal vision statement in the aftermath of loss is a journey of deep self-reflection and future-forward thinking. It's about rediscovering who you are and what you aspire to be in the wake of a life-altering tragedy. Here's how you can embark on this transformative process:

1. **Engage in Deep Self-Reflection:** This is the first and most crucial step. Reflect on your core values, beliefs, and aspirations. What drives you? What are your passions? Consider the aspects of life that give you a sense of purpose and fulfillment.

2. **Visualize a Future Beyond Grief:** Allow yourself to envision a future that exists within your new reality. What does this future look like? How does it align with your core values and the legacy you wish to leave?

3. **Embrace Authenticity:** Your vision statement should be a genuine representation of your true self. It's important to be honest and authentic in this process, even if it means facing uncomfortable truths or unexplored aspirations.

4. **Craft a Clear and Concise Statement:** A vision statement should be succinct yet powerful. Use clear, positive language to articulate your vision. This statement should encapsulate your aspirations and serve as a constant reminder of your path forward. As an example, here's my own vision statement:

My best days are still ahead. My best laughs, my best smile, my best meal, my best trip, my best kiss, my best hug, my best sunrise, my best sleep, my best celebration is still ahead. My marriage is filled with love, passion, giving, and romance. My relationship with my daughter continues to grow stronger as Ava grows into a strong and beautiful woman. I am thankful and honor the life of my son, Alexander. I am healthy and abundant, full of life and vigor. I am strong and courageous and well equipped for the challenges of today. Above all else, I am filled with gratitude for all that I have experienced, and all I will experience in the days to come.

5. **Integrate Both Passion and Purpose:** Your vision statement should resonate with what truly excites and scares you a little. It should connect to your higher source of unlimited power and potential.

6. **Align with Your Goals:** Make sure your vision statement aligns with your immediate and long-term goals. This alignment strengthens the purpose and importance of your vision.

7. **Commit to Your Vision:** A vision statement is not just words on paper; it's a commitment to a new way of living. Regularly review and recite your vision statement to embed it into your daily life.

8. **Stay Flexible and Open to Revision:** As you grow and evolve, so too should your vision statement. Be open to making adjustments as you gain new insights and experiences.

The Impact of a Vision Statement on Healing

The power of a vision statement in the healing process cannot be overstated. It provides a sense of direction and hope during a time when both can feel lost. It's a tool for recalibrating your life's trajectory, helping you to navigate through the fog of grief and emerge with a renewed sense of purpose.

Regularly engaging with your vision statement can transform your outlook on life. It shifts your focus from the pain of the present to the potential of the future, instilling a sense of optimism and motivation. This shift doesn't negate the pain of your loss but offers a way to live with it, integrating it into a broader narrative of growth and resilience.

THE POWER OF BREATHING

In the labyrinth of grief, where every breath can feel like a struggle, the discovery of the power of breathing was akin to finding an oasis in a desert. The simple act of breathing, often taken for granted, became a lifeline in the darkest moments of my journey.

In the raw aftermath of my loss, I noticed how my breathing patterns had changed. The deep, rhythmic breaths I once took without thought were replaced by shallow gasps, as if my body was in a constant state of shock, fighting for emotional survival. This struggle with breath became a physical manifestation of my internal turmoil, a relentless reminder of the pain that clung to my heart.

One night, my breathing became so labored it felt as though I was suffocating under the immense burden of my grief. Almost instinctively, I began practicing what I later learned was called controlled breathing, specifically, the "box-breathing" technique. This is how it worked.

Sitting up in the darkness of my room, I began to consciously guide my breath, inhaling, holding, exhaling, and pausing, each for a count of four. The effect was immediate and profound. With each cycle, a sense of calm began to wash over me, steadying my heart and clearing the fog that had settled in my mind.

Emboldened by this experience, I delved deeper into the world of breathing techniques, integrating them into my daily routine. Each method offered its unique form of solace, from deep belly breathing to more structured practices. The discipline of guiding my breath became not just a tool for moments of panic but a daily ritual to center myself in the present, providing a brief respite from the relentless tide of grief.

Physical and Mental Benefits of Controlled Breathing

1. **Stress Reduction:** Controlled breathing is a powerful ally in reducing stress. It activates the body's relaxation response, helping to lower heart rate and blood pressure, and release muscle tension.

2. **Enhanced Respiratory Function:** Regular practice of breathing exercises can improve lung capacity and efficiency, making each breath more effective and easing the physical strain often experienced during intense emotional stress.

3. **Pain Management:** For those experiencing physical pain, whether due to grief-induced tension or other causes, focused breathing can provide a natural form of pain relief, easing discomfort through relaxation and distraction. (Women have been using belly breathing and pant-pant-blow techniques during childbirth for centuries.)

4. **Improved Sleep:** As grief often disrupts sleep patterns, incorporating breathing exercises into your nightly routine can significantly enhance the quality of your rest, facilitating a more peaceful and restorative sleep.

5. **Emotional Regulation:** Controlled breathing plays a crucial role in managing emotions. It helps to calm the nervous system, reducing feelings of anxiety and helping to stabilize mood swings often associated with grief.

To reap the benefits of controlled breathing, consider incorporating it into your daily routine. Here are some general tips to get started:

1. **Create a Calm Environment:** Find a quiet space where you can practice without distractions. A peaceful setting can enhance the effectiveness of your breathing exercises.

2. **Adopt a Comfortable Posture:** Whether you choose to sit or lie down, ensure your posture supports easy breathing. A straight, relaxed spine is key to allowing unrestricted airflow.

3. **Focus on Your Breath:** Pay attention to the rhythm of your breathing. Notice the sensation of air entering and leaving your body. Aim to make each breath deep and steady.

4. **Experiment with Techniques:** Try different breathing methods to find what works best for you. The 4-7-8 technique, deep belly breathing, and alternate nostril breathing are all excellent places to start. (Just Google or check YouTube for how-tos.)

5. **Be Consistent:** Like any practice, the benefits of controlled breathing are most pronounced with regular practice. Set aside a few minutes each day to focus on your breath.

6. **Use Guided Sessions:** If you're new to breathing exercises, consider using guided sessions from apps or online videos. They can provide valuable instructions and help you to maintain focus.

Through the simple yet profound act of controlled breathing, I found a way to navigate the tumultuous waves of grief. It became a daily ritual, a moment of stillness in a sea of chaos, an

MORE HEALING AHEAD

As I journeyed through the transformative practices of sweat and the grounding power of a vision statement, augmented by the subtle yet profound art of controlled breathing, I found not just solace, but a roadmap for navigating the treacherous terrain of grief.

These therapies, each unique, collectively provided a foundation for healing, revealing to me the untapped reservoirs of strength and resilience within. With each run, each breath and each reiteration of my vision statement, I discovered that there were more layers to uncover, more ways to not only cope with grief but to transform it into a force for positive change in my life. As I ventured forward, I found additional therapies that would continue to shape my path towards recovery and personal growth.

Chapter 10:

THERAPIES FOR HEALING, PART 2

Combating Hopelessness

As I began to integrate the practices of sweat, vision, and controlled breathing into my daily life, a subtle yet significant shift occurred in my journey through grief. The pain and sorrow, ever-present companions in my heart, didn't vanish, but I started to encounter them with a newfound fortitude.

The once overwhelming enemies in the arena of my mind began to lose some of their power, overshadowed by a growing sense of hope. This change, although gradual, fueled my resolve to delve deeper into additional healing techniques. I realized that each therapy I embraced not only equipped me to face my grief but also to actively engage in combat with the adversaries of despair and hopelessness.

THE POWER OF MEDITATION

Among these newfound tools, the power of meditation emerged as a critical ally, a way to reshape my internal world and reinforce the strength I was slowly reclaiming. This ancient practice, rooted in the art of focusing attention and clearing the mind, became a beacon of tranquility in the tumultuous sea of grief.

Embracing Meditation in the Midst of Grief

My initial experiences with meditation were marked by apprehension. The concept, shrouded in mystery, seemed distant from my world of tangible grief and loss. However, as the chaotic storm of thoughts and emotions intensified, the need for an anchor became apparent. Meditation, with its promise of inner peace and self-awareness, beckoned me towards a journey of mindfulness.

The early days of this journey were challenging. My mind, a battlefield of relentless memories and "what ifs," struggled to embrace the stillness meditation required. Yet, with each attempt, I found a gradual easing of the internal turmoil. Combining techniques that I was already using like box breathing with guided meditations offered structured pathways to regain control over my thoughts and emotions.

The Transformative Power of Meditation

Meditation offers a respite from the tumultuous waves of emotion that grief brings. It allows you to center yourself, to find calm within the storm. By focusing on your breath, or engaging in guided meditations, you create a space where healing can begin. This quiet introspection enables you to process your emotions at a pace that feels right for you.

Meditation is not just about quieting the mind; it's about opening the heart. It's a practice that nurtures resilience and fosters a deep sense of connection to something greater than oneself. As meditation becomes a regular practice, its transformative power unfolds. It shifts your perspective, allowing you to view your pain and grief through a lens of compassion and understanding. You'll find moments of profound insight and peace that can light your path through the darkest times as you experience the following physical and mental benefits.

1. **Stress Reduction:** Meditation significantly lowers stress levels. By calming the mind and body, it reduces the production of stress hormones, creating a sense of overall well-being.

2. **Improved Respiratory Health:** Breath-focused meditation enhances lung function, increasing oxygen flow to the brain and body, which is crucial for healing and recovery.

3. **Pain Management:** Focusing on breath and mindfulness during meditation can help in managing physical pain, a common companion of intense emotional grief.

4. **Improved Sleep Quality:** Meditation aids in alleviating sleep disturbances, a common issue during periods of grief. It promotes relaxation, leading to deeper and more restorative sleep.

5. **Emotional Regulation:** Regular meditation practice is key in managing emotions. It fosters emotional stability, helping to balance the highs and lows experienced in grief.

6. **Increased Self-awareness:** Meditation deepens self-awareness, allowing a greater understanding of personal emotions, thoughts, and behaviors, which is essential in the journey of healing and personal growth.

7. **Enhanced Concentration and Creativity:** Meditation improves focus and clears the mind, fostering creativity and better decision-making, which can often be clouded by grief.

8. **Spiritual Connection:** Meditation fosters a deep connection to one's spirituality, providing a sense of peace and clarity amidst the chaos of loss and pain. Whether it's connecting with a higher power, the universe, or your inner self, meditation can be a profoundly spiritual experience. It invites tranquility and a sense of oneness with a greater existence, offering comfort and reassurance.

Incorporating Meditation Into Daily Life

Adopting meditation as a part of my daily routine was transformative. It required setting realistic expectations, finding a quiet space, and committing to a regular practice. Guided meditations were particularly helpful in the beginning, providing structure and focus.

Incorporating meditation into your daily routine need not be daunting. Start with just a few minutes each day, gradually increasing the time as you become more comfortable. Find a quiet space where you won't be disturbed. You may choose to focus on your breath, use a mantra, or follow guided meditations. The key is consistency and allowing yourself the grace to experience this journey without judgment.

Over time, I learned to embrace the wandering of my mind during meditation, gently guiding it back to the present moment. Consistency in practice proved more crucial than the duration of each session. Gradually, meditation became not just a practice but a sanctuary, a place of peace and resilience amidst life's storms.

THE POWER OF JOURNALING

Journaling is perhaps the most intimate form of self-expression. It invites an unfiltered exploration of one's inner world, revealing layers of complexity in our thoughts and emotions. The act of transferring thoughts to paper can be incredibly liberating, a tangible release of the turmoil within.

Journaling has been a part of my life for as long as I can remember. It has served as a companion through the undulations of life, capturing my thoughts, emotions, and experiences. Reflecting on past entries, I've often found a blend of pride and amusement at my younger self's musings. Each entry stands as a testament to who I was at that moment, a snapshot of my evolving self.

However, journaling took on a new dimension as I navigated the depths of grief. On countless sleepless nights, my journal became the vessel into which I poured my soul. Initially, the pages were filled with raw emotions—anger, regret, and an endless stream of questions. It was a tumultuous period, but journaling offered a unique perspective, allowing me to track the evolution of my thoughts and feelings over time. Some entries were marked by progress, others by setbacks, but together, they painted a picture of resilience and strength I hadn't realized I possessed.

Benefits of Journaling in Healing

1. **Stress Reduction:** Writing about our innermost thoughts and feelings can significantly lower stress levels, providing a much-needed emotional outlet.

2. **Self-Reflection and Awareness:** Journaling fosters a deeper understanding of oneself. It helps in identifying patterns in thoughts and behaviors, contributing to personal growth.

3. **Navigating Emotion:** Putting your feelings on paper serves as a safe space to navigate complex emotions associated with grief, providing a sense of clarity and understanding.

4. **Problem Solving and Decision Making:** Journaling can clarify thoughts, aiding in problem solving and decision making.

5. **Memory Preservation:** Journals act as keepers of memories, chronicling life experiences that shape who we are.

6. **Enhancing Communication Skills:** Regular journaling improves writing and articulation skills, benefiting personal and professional communication.

7. **Creative Exploration:** For those inclined toward creativity, journaling is an avenue for artistic expression and exploration of new ideas.

8. **Positive Outlook:** Maintaining a gratitude journal can shift focus to positive aspects of life, enhancing overall well-being.

Incorporating Journaling Into Daily Life

Journaling became a daily ritual for me. Whether reflecting on the past, envisioning the future, or anchoring in the present, the act of writing brought clarity and peace. If you want to start a journal, here are some tips:

1. **Choose Your Medium:** Whether a traditional notebook or a digital app, select a journaling medium that resonates with you.

2. **Create a Routine:** Dedicate a specific time each day to write in your journal. Consistency enhances the benefits.

3. **Write Freely:** Let your thoughts flow without censorship. The journal is a judgment-free zone.

4. **Focus on Feelings:** Express your emotions openly. Journaling is a tool for emotional exploration and understanding.

5. **Use Prompts:** Journaling has the power to connect the emotions and stirrings of the soul with our conscious minds, so that we can let it breathe, release, and in some cases, question the bias or incorrect story that may be causing pain. If you're unsure where to start, use prompts like these to describe what you're feeling right now:

   - Why is that important or why does it matter?
   - What is the story I'm telling myself and is it helping or hurting me?
   - If the story is causing me pain, is it true or am I adding a bias?
   - In light of what or who may be missing, what am I truly grateful for right now?

6. **Reflect and Grow:** Regularly review your entries. This reflection can offer insights into your personal growth journey.

Journaling was more than a mere pastime; it became a crucial part of my healing process. It allowed me to confront my grief, to understand it, and eventually, to weave it into the fabric of my life. In sharing my journaling journey, I hope to inspire you to discover the power of your own written word as a tool for healing, self-discovery, and transformation.

THE POWER OF SELF-TALK

The transformative journey of grief introduced me to the profound impact of self-talk. This internal monologue, a constant companion, can be our greatest ally or our most critical adversary.

In the aftermath of my son's passing, I grappled with the darker aspects of self-talk. This voice became a relentless critic, echoing my deepest insecurities and fears, constantly reminding me of my perceived failures as a father and individual.

The relentless barrage of negative self-talk amplified my grief, leading me into depths of depression. It was an inescapable presence, coloring every moment of my existence with a hue of despair. This realization led me to a pivotal decision: to take control of this inner narrative. I began to actively engage with these self-deprecating thoughts, challenging them, and seeking to transform them into affirmations of self-worth and resilience.

Positive Self-Talk as a Healing Dialogue

The conversations we have with ourselves shape our perception of reality. Negative self-talk can trap us in a cycle of despair, reinforcing feelings of hopelessness and inadequacy. In contrast, positive self-talk acts as a beacon of hope. It involves consciously shifting our internal dialogue from criticism and self-doubt to affirmation and self-compassion. This shift doesn't happen overnight; it requires persistence and patience. But the impact is profound—a transformed mindset leads to a life experienced through a lens of possibility and strength.

Gradually, the tone of my inner voice began to change. The journey was slow, marked by setbacks and moments of doubt, but the trajectory was unmistakably positive. I started to notice moments of peace, clarity, and even joy. This shift in self-talk not only alleviated my grief but began to reshape my entire outlook on life.

Benefits of Positive Self-Talk

1. **Improved Mental Health:** The shift from negative to positive self-talk significantly reduced my anxiety and depression, replacing despair with hope.

2. **Increased Self-Esteem:** Positive self-talk fostered a sense of self-worth and confidence, crucial in the process of healing and personal growth.

3.   **Better Decision Making:** With a clearer, more positive mindset, I found myself making decisions that were more aligned with my true values and aspirations.

4.   **Enhanced Relationships:** As my self-talk improved, so did my relationships. I became more open, empathetic, and connected with those around me.

5.   **Resilience in Adversity:** Positive self-talk equipped me with the resilience to face life's challenges, transforming obstacles into opportunities for growth.

Embracing a New Narrative

To reshape my self-talk, I started by journaling the negative thoughts, confronting them head-on, and questioning their validity. Would I ever speak to a loved one in such a harsh manner? Certainly not.

This exercise in self-awareness was the first step in changing the narrative. I began to counter each negative thought with a positive affirmation, a statement of self-love and acceptance.

Today, my self-talk is a source of comfort, guidance, and encouragement. It's a testament to the power of the mind to heal and transform even in the face of the deepest grief. This journey has taught me that the voice inside our head can be our most powerful tool in overcoming adversity, a constant reminder of our inherent worth and resilience.

To anyone struggling with negative self-talk, especially in the face of grief, I offer this advice: be relentless in challenging those inner criticisms. Replace each negative thought with a positive affirmation. It may feel forced at first, but with time and persistence, this practice can transform your internal dialogue into a source of strength and empowerment.

THE POWER OF DAILY GOAL SETTING

In the arena of my grief the power of daily goal setting became another potent weapon against despair. This practice, seemingly simple yet profound, became a beacon of light in the darkest corners of my mind.

As I navigated through the fog of loss, the concept of time transformed. Hours stretched into what seemed like endless days, each moment a relentless reminder of my son's absence. In this altered reality, setting daily goals emerged as anchors—firm points of focus in the turbulent sea of my emotions.

I began with small, manageable goals. It started as simple as making the bed, then progressed to tasks like taking a walk or spending focused time with my daughter. These goals, though modest, were monumental in their significance. They were acts of defiance against the inertia of grief, small victories in a larger battle for recovery.

Each completed goal sent ripples through the stagnant waters of my grief. With every achievement, no matter how minor, a sense of accomplishment pierced through the haze of sorrow. It was a reminder that despite the overwhelming sense of loss, I was still capable of still moving forward, step by small step.

This practice of setting daily goals evolved into a ritual, a sacred time each morning where I would sit with my thoughts and chart out my day. This ritual became a space of reflection and intention, where I could align my actions with my deeper purpose and desires.

Goal Setting as a Pathway to Healing

The act of daily goal setting transcended mere task completion. It became a pathway to healing, a method to rebuild the fractured pieces of my identity. In each goal, I found fragments of the person I used to be and glimpses of the person I aspired to become.

The goals varied, from physical activities like running and yoga, to emotional and spiritual practices like meditation and journaling. Each goal was a step towards a holistic healing journey, addressing not just the mind or body but the entirety of my being.

As I look back on those early days of setting goals, I see them as the first rays of a new dawn. They were the initial steps on a long road to recovery, a road marked by both triumphs and setbacks. But with each goal set and achieved, I reclaimed a piece of myself, and in doing so, edged closer to a life defined not by loss, but by love, purpose, and resilience.

In the arena of grief, armed with the power of daily goal setting I found not just a way to survive, but a way to thrive. For anyone walking this path, know this: small steps lead to great journeys, and in the tapestry of grief, every thread counts. Your goals, your commitments, all matter. They are the building blocks of your healing, the foundation of a future forged with purpose and hope.

THE POWER OF INTEGRITY

In the midst of grief's arena, where the specters of loss and despair loomed, I discovered another vital tool in my arsenal: the power of integrity. This wasn't just about honesty or moral uprightness; it was about wholeness, about being undivided in the face of life's harshest trials. Integrity became the glue that bound my actions to my values, the force that held me accountable to myself and my journey.

In this newfound understanding of integrity, I found a deeper resolve to honor my commitments, not just to others, but most importantly, to myself. Each goal, each day, was a promise I made to myself—a promise to keep moving, to keep fighting, to keep living.

Integrity: The Unseen Shield

As I navigated the labyrinth of my sorrow, I found that integrity acted as an unseen shield, guarding not just my actions but the very essence of who I was. In the early days of my grief, when I felt fragmented and lost, integrity helped me hold the pieces together. It became a guiding principle, a north star that kept me true to myself and my values, even when everything else was in disarray.

One of the greatest challenges I faced was maintaining consistency in my actions and decisions. Grief has a way of clouding judgment, of making you question your beliefs and values. But through the lens of integrity, I strived to remain consistent and to make decisions that aligned with my core values, even when they were difficult or painful.

Integrity in grief meant allowing myself to fully experience the depths of my emotions without losing sight of who I was. It meant giving myself permission to weep, to mourn, and to be vulnerable, yet also to rise, to rebuild, and to find moments of joy without guilt. It was a delicate balancing act, one that required constant self-reflection and adjustment.

Integrity as Self-Care

I learned that living with integrity was a form of self-care. It was about honoring my commitments to myself, about respecting my own needs and boundaries. This included setting aside time for meditation, exercise, and journaling. It was about saying no when I needed to and yes to things that aligned with my healing journey.

I realized that integrity was about the wholeness of being. It was about integrating all aspects of myself—the grieving father, the husband, the friend, the professional—into a cohesive whole. It was about understanding that all these roles were facets of the same diamond, each reflecting a different part of my identity.

Integrity shaped my path through grief. It was the thread that connected each step, each therapy, each moment of breakthrough and setback. Integrity kept me grounded when the world seemed to shift beneath my feet. It was a reminder that even in the heart of darkness, I could be whole, I could be true to myself, and I could emerge stronger.

For anyone walking the path of grief, know this: integrity is your ally. It is the quiet strength that sustains you when all else fails. In the tapestry of your journey, let integrity be the thread that binds, that holds, that weaves a story of resilience, hope, and enduring love.

Chapter 11:

PRACTICES FOR TRANSFORMATION AND EMPOWERMENT

The Will to Survive and Thrive

As I fled through the darkened arena of my grief, pursued by monstrous creatures born of my deepest fears, the ground beneath me suddenly gave way and I fell into an unexpected haven in the midst of chaos. Away from their relentless pursuit, I caught my breath. As I gathered my senses, my eyes fell upon an unassuming, dust-covered box. It seemed out of place in this grim place, yet it called to me with a silent promise of hope.

Cautiously, I approached the box. Inside I discovered an array of tools, each representing one of the healing therapies I had embraced—embodiments of sweat, vision, self-talk, meditation, and more. Beside the box lay a journal, its leather cover worn from use, a testament to my journey filled with the echoes of my heartache, struggles, and resilience.

In that moment, a profound sense of relief washed over me. These weren't just tools for coping; they were weapons in my fight against despair, tangible symbols of my struggle to reclaim my life from the jaws of grief.

I allowed myself a moment to feel the full weight of my emotions—the pain, the loss, and the exhaustion—and also a burgeoning sense of hope and strength. I realized that, despite everything, I was still standing, still fighting. These tools were more than mere aids; they were extensions of my will to survive and thrive.

With the journal in my hand, I felt a newfound resolve take root. I was battered and weary yet not defeated. Each tool in that box was a step towards healing, a way to face the beasts above me with newfound resilience and courage.

Ready to re-enter the fray, I returned to the arena where the monstrous creatures that had once seemed invincible now appeared less formidable. I understood that the battle was far from over, but I now felt equipped to face it head-on. I was weary, yes, but also hopeful—hopeful that with each step forward, each therapy embraced, each word penned, I was moving closer to mastering the enemies that once sought to destroy me.

This was no longer just a tale of survival; it was a story of transformation and empowerment. A man, once consumed by grief, now stood ready to shape his future, one breath, one thought, one day at a time.

***

CRAFTING A PERSONALIZED STRATEGY FOR HEALING AND GROWTH

I'm grateful that you've accompanied me this far on a journey that, for me, has been nothing short of a fight for survival. It's been a matter of life and death, a battle to reclaim the essence of who I am. The tools and therapies we've explored together possess the remarkable potential to transform lives, to offer a way to rise triumphantly from the depths of despair. I'm convinced that without them, my life would be unrecognizable, a mere shadow of its former self. These aren't just abstract concepts; they're lifelines that have anchored me in my darkest hours.

The journey of healing and transformation isn't about the obstacles becoming easier; it's about becoming stronger, more resilient. I'm confident that you, too, can harness this strength. By learning how to effectively incorporate these therapies into your life, you can confront and overcome the beasts that lurk in the arena of your own life.

In the struggle against the multifaceted nature of grief, it's important to recognize that different aspects of our pain respond to different therapeutic approaches. Each therapy has its unique strengths; but when synergized, they create a formidable force against the internal battles we face. By understanding how to match specific therapies to particular "enemies," we can effectively disarm the power they hold over us.

Targeting Hopelessness with Vision Statements and Goal Setting

Hopelessness often stems from a loss of direction and purpose. By crafting vision statements and setting daily goals, you can reorient your focus towards the future. These tools help you to envision a life beyond grief, restoring hope by mapping out achievable steps towards a fulfilling purpose.

Countering Guilt and Negative Self-Talk with Positive Self-Talk and Journaling

The enemy of guilt and a harsh internal critic can be silenced through positive self-talk and journaling. By actively rewriting your internal dialogue and recording your thoughts and feelings, you transform guilt into self-compassion and negative judgments into affirmations of your worth and capabilities.

Dissolving Anger Through Integrity and Physical Exercise

Physical exercise serves as a healthy outlet for anger, allowing you to channel intense emotions into physical activity. Coupled with living a life of integrity, where actions align with values, exercise can help in processing and releasing anger in a way that is constructive rather than destructive.

Alleviating Detachment from Reality with Meditation and Mindfulness

Detachment from reality, a form of escapism from pain, can be addressed through meditation and mindfulness. These practices ground you in the present moment, fostering a sense of connection to the here and now and help to anchor you in reality.

Confronting Nihilism with a Blend of Vision, Meditation, and Positive Actions

Nihilism, the sense that nothing matters, is perhaps the most insidious enemy. Combating it requires a combination of vision for the future, the clarity gained from meditation, and taking positive actions. Together, these practices reinforce the belief in life's meaning and your role in shaping it.

ACCELERATING HEALING THROUGH THERAPEUTIC PRACTICES

The journey through grief and the battle against its accompanying enemies is not a passive process. Active engagement with therapeutic practices can significantly accelerate healing, reducing the time you are held in the grip of emotional turmoil.

Combining and implementing these therapeutic tools into daily life isn't just about coping; it's about transformation. Each practice, from physical exercise to meditation, serves not only to alleviate immediate pain but also to rebuild and to strengthen you from within.

Exercise and Self-Talk: When combined, these practices not only improve physical health but also reshape mental narratives. They empower you to combat negative thoughts and reinforce a positive self-image, crucial in navigating the path of grief. The physical exertion of exercise provides a tangible outlet for emotional tension, while positive self-talk reinforces the mental fortitude to persevere.

To integrate these therapies effectively, start by setting realistic and achievable goals for physical activity. It could be as simple as a daily walk or a set number of steps. Pair this physical activity with intentional positive affirmations. For example, while on a walk, you might repeat affirmations such as "I am strong," "I am capable," or "I am healing." This practice aligns the body and mind in a dance of recovery and empowerment.

Meditation and Mindfulness: Regular meditation enhances mental clarity and emotional balance. Mindfulness keeps you grounded in the present, preventing you from being overwhelmed by past regrets or future anxieties.

For meditation and mindfulness, which are great for improving mental clarity and emotional balance, you might find it helpful to carve out a special time each day for this practice. How about in the mornings or just before bed? Aim for around 10 to 20 minutes where you can really focus on your breath and being in the moment. There are plenty of guided meditations available online, especially on YouTube, that are tailored for healing and acceptance. This routine can really ground you, helping to keep those overwhelming thoughts about the past or future at bay.

Vision Statements and Goal Setting: These tools provide a roadmap for the future, an essential component for anyone who feels lost in the aftermath of a tragedy. They help you to set and achieve small, manageable goals, gradually leading to larger accomplishments and a renewed sense of purpose.

To effectively blend vision statements with daily goal setting, aim to align your everyday activities directly with the broader vision you have for your life. For instance, if your vision statement includes being physically and mentally prepared for life's challenges to fully enjoy moments with your children, then your daily goals should reflect this intention. A practical daily goal could be engaging in a 30-minute cardio workout each morning, which contributes to your fitness and overall health. Following this, spending quality active time with your children, like playing tag at the park, directly ties into your vision of cherishing moments with them. This approach ensures that your day-to-day actions are woven into the larger fabric of your life's aspirations, creating a cohesive and fulfilling journey towards your envisioned future.

Journaling: This practice offers a safe space for emotional expression and reflection, crucial for processing and understanding your grief journey.

Integrating journaling with other therapeutic practices enhances its benefits. For instance, after engaging in a meditation and mindfulness session, you could journal about the experience, noting the peace and clarity it brought you, perhaps feelings reminiscent of childhood serenity. This reflection helps solidify the benefits of the practice and gives you tangible evidence of its impact.

Similarly, if you're working on positive self-talk, journaling can be a space to explore its effects. You might write about how morning affirmations set a positive tone for your day and how this shift in mindset positively influenced an afternoon meeting with friends. By documenting these experiences, you not only track your progress but also deepen your understanding of how each therapeutic practice contributes to your overall well-being

Living with Integrity: This underpins all other practices. By aligning your actions with your values and commitments, you cultivate a sense of self-respect and purpose that supports all other healing efforts.

Living with integrity involves consciously choosing to align your daily actions with your core values and long-term goals. This alignment fosters a life of purpose and authenticity. To practice integrity, consider conducting regular value alignment checks. This means taking time to reflect on your daily decisions and actions to ensure they are in harmony with your fundamental beliefs and objectives. It's like a personal audit that keeps you true to your path and principles.

Additionally, setting reminders or establishing rituals can serve as powerful tools to reinforce your commitments, both to yourself and to others. These practices act as constant cues, reminding you of the importance of maintaining your integrity, which in turn, nurtures your self-worth and solidifies your character. Through these actions, you actively cultivate a life that not only reflects your values but also enhances your sense of purpose and fulfillment.

By integrating these practices into your daily routine, you create a holistic approach to healing. This approach not only addresses the symptoms of grief but also fosters growth, resilience, and a deeper understanding of self. The journey might be challenging, but the transformation it brings can lead to a renewed sense of strength and purpose.

REFLECTING ON THE HEALING JOURNEY

As you journey through the process of grief, taking a moment to reflect on the path you've traveled can be profoundly enlightening. Reflection allows you to acknowledge the progress you've made, even if it doesn't always feel like it.

Looking back, you may realize that the intensity of your pain has lessened over time, that moments of joy have started to seep back into your life. You might notice that the therapies you've implemented have not only helped you manage grief but also brought about personal growth and self-discovery.

Realizing the Impact of Therapies: When you first started using these tools, they might have seemed like mere survival tactics. But over time, their deeper impact becomes apparent. The physical strength gained from exercise, the mental clarity from meditation, the emotional release from journaling, and the resilience from positive self-talk, all converge to create a stronger, more centered version of you.

Growth and Transformation: Grief is not a journey you would have chosen, but within it lies the potential for profound transformation. Through coping and healing, you develop qualities like empathy, resilience, and a deeper appreciation for life.

From Surviving to Thriving: The ultimate goal of this journey is not just to survive grief but to reach a place where you can thrive again. This doesn't mean forgetting or completely overcoming the pain but finding a way to live with it, allowing it to be part of your story, not the entirety of it.

This period of reflection is not just about looking back but also about looking forward. It's about recognizing that while grief may always be a part of you, it doesn't have to define you. As you continue to use these tools and therapies, you pave the way for a future that, while different from what you might have envisioned, can still be filled with hope, purpose, and joy.

ENCOURAGING ADOPTION OF THERAPIES

Healing is not a linear process, and maintaining the gains made requires ongoing effort and commitment. One way to continue practicing the various therapies we've explored here is to encourage and to help others who might be navigating similar paths of grief and loss to adopt them as part of their healing process, too.

The journey through grief is not a solitary one. By encouraging the adoption of therapeutic practices, you not only continue to heal yourself but also extend a hand to others. This collective journey of healing can foster a community of resilience, understanding, and compassion.

Universal Application: While your journey is unique, the tools and techniques you've utilized have universal applicability. Others may find solace and strength in these same practices. Encourage those around you who are struggling with grief or emotional turmoil to consider adopting some of these therapies.

Sharing Your Story: One of the most powerful ways to encourage others is by sharing your story. Your experiences, the challenges you faced, and the strategies that helped you can provide a roadmap for others. It also helps to humanize the process, showing that while grief is deeply personal, it is also a shared human experience.

Support and Community: Building a support system or joining a community of individuals who are also on their healing journey can be incredibly beneficial. It provides a space to share experiences, to offer and receive encouragement, and to remind each other that no one is alone in their struggle.

Customization and Adaptation: Remind others that it's okay to customize and adapt these practices to fit their unique circumstances and needs. Encouraging experimentation and personalization can help individuals find what works best for them.

Advocating for Mental Health: Part of encouraging the adoption of these therapies involves advocating for mental health awareness and the de-stigmatization of seeking help. Promoting an environment where emotional well-being is prioritized can pave the way for more people to seek the support they need. (I've provided some resources for anyone facing an immediate crisis at the end of this book.)

In the spirit of fostering mental health awareness and breaking down the barriers of stigma, I am proud to share the mission of the Xan You Matter Foundation, an initiative that Debra and I hold close to our hearts. This foundation emerged from our own journey through the valleys of depression, anxiety, and the shadow of suicidal thoughts, dedicated to offering a lifeline to those who find themselves in similar struggles. Our commitment is to provide support, education, and resources, aiming to kindle hope, spread awareness, and dismantle the stigma surrounding mental health issues.

If this journey resonates with you, if you feel the stirrings of a desire to reach out for support or to stand with us in this cause, I warmly invite you to connect. Details on how to get in touch with the Xan You Matter Foundation, to seek help, or to join us as a volunteer are waiting for you at the end of this book. Your voice, your hand, your heart can contribute to the wave of change we are passionately driving forward. Together, we affirm the value of every life and we stand united in the belief that it's never too late to reach out—because there is hope and every life truly matters.

Chapter 12:

SURRENDER

———

The Call of the Hairpins

It was a brisk December evening in 2020. Over a year had passed since my son's suicide and the beginning of my journey through the crucible of grief.

Cruising down a familiar road on my motorcycle, my grief felt like a clamp around my chest. The landscape around me blurred into a backdrop for my inner storm. Anger and despair dominated my being, a stark contrast to the serenity of the setting sun. As darkness engulfed me outside, inside a hurricane of emotions raged, growing in intensity. My world seemed to be collapsing, and my thoughts spiraled chaotically, mirroring the tumultuous path of my motorcycle.

The darkness wasn't just a lack of light; it was a canvas for my inner demons to manifest. Despair, hopelessness, and a destructive form of nihilism—the metaphorical monsters of my personal arena—surrounded and overwhelmed me, seemingly as real as the cool desert air against my skin. Fueled by the intense emotions coursing through me, I toyed with the idea that a simple veer to the left, a deliberate plunge off the road into the abyss, could end it all. I balanced on the razor's edge between life and reckless abandon, consumed by the rawest form of despair in a desperate dance with danger, flirting with finality.

As I navigated each hairpin turn, the curves whispered seductive yet sinister invitations, beckoning me to abandon the world I knew, to reunite with my son who had departed too soon. The speed of my motorcycle matched the racing of my heart, both seemingly beyond my control. I was consumed by an intense longing to be with my son, believing there was nothing left for me in a world he no longer inhabited.

In the chaos of my thoughts, the voices in my head grew into a deafening scream, impossible to ignore, each turn in the road amplifying their call, invisible hands tugging at me, luring me deeper into the darkness. But then, amidst this tumultuous symphony of despair, a solitary, soft voice emerged, cutting through the haunting chorus with its gentle yet piercing clarity.

"What about Ava? What about Debra?" it whispered. "Doesn't Ava need her father? Doesn't Debra need her husband?"

This voice brought with it a profound realization: my presence was crucial for the ones I loved. It asked me to consider who would protect them from their demons, from the challenges and grief they would face if I succumbed to mine. It was a crucial reminder that my journey was not just about me, but also about those I held dear.

Summoning every ounce of strength I had left, I began the Herculean task of easing off the accelerator. As I slowed down, the wind's intensity lessened, and I came to a complete stop. In the stillness, I allowed myself to fully feel the weight of my emotions. I wept uncontrollably, releasing the pent-up anguish and fear that had been gripping me.

In that vulnerable state, I realized how close I had come to succumbing to the ultimate goal of my metaphorical monsters. The symbols of my grief and despair had been tearing at me, piece by piece, driving me toward a state of living death. Their aim was clear: to wear me down until I could no longer stand, until they could consume my very soul.

This moment of realization marked a profound turning point

in my journey. It was not only a raw confrontation with the depths of my despair but a crucial awakening to the resilience within me. I understood then that surrendering to these forces would not only be giving up on myself but also on those who needed me. This encounter with the edge of oblivion became a catalyst, propelling me towards a path of healing and, ultimately, surrender in its truest, most life-affirming form.

**

THE DAWN OF SURRENDER

The morning after that harrowing experience, I made a decision that would mark the beginning of true change in my life. Recognizing the gravity of what had almost transpired, I checked myself into a mental health facility for a week-long observation. That call to the void had been alarmingly close, nearly stripping everything away from me. In that moment of clarity, I understood the necessity of seeking assistance; it was imperative if I was to emerge victorious from this battle.

This step represented my first genuine act of surrender, a surrender to the concept of receiving help, an acceptance of the journey ahead. It signified a surrender to the process of healing, a recognition that life as I knew it had irreversibly changed and that I needed support to navigate this new reality.

Admitting the need for help was a crucial turning point. It was an acknowledgment that the poison of grief and despair within me needed to be addressed professionally. This was not about admitting defeat; rather, it was about embracing the strength that comes from knowing when to seek guidance and support. It was a step towards dismantling the harmful notions I held about self-reliance in the face of overwhelming emotional turmoil.

In this act of surrender, there was power and hope. It marked the beginning of a journey towards healing, towards understanding that while the path ahead would be challenging, it was not one I had to walk alone. This realization was a pivotal moment in my journey, one that would lay the groundwork for the transformation and peace I was striving to achieve.

A CATALYST FOR CHANGE

During my stay within the tranquility and structured environment of the mental health facility, I met many young people who were navigating their own crises on the path to recovery and whose struggles mirrored my son's. I saw in them a reflection of the battle my son had faced—a battle I, too, was fervently fighting. This realization ignited a remarkable transformation in me, awakening the protector, the nurturer, the father I had always been to my children. It also rekindled the leadership qualities I exhibited with my coworkers, whom I had always regarded as an extended family.

Watching and listening to their stories about confronting the same deceptive and destructive forces that had nearly overwhelmed me filled my heart with a newfound purpose. It was a stark reminder that the enemies of despair and hopelessness were not just personal adversaries; they were universal, preying on countless others, particularly our youth.

This revelation was yet another turning point. It reawakened my fighting spirit, not just for my own life, but for the lives of those around me—my family, who still needed me, and the broader community that was silently battling similar demons. I realized that my journey was far from over; it was evolving into something greater. I was not only fighting for my own recovery but also for those who needed guidance and support, those who might benefit from the hard-earned lessons of my own struggles.

This shift in perspective marked a significant step in my journey of surrender. It was no longer just about surrendering to the process of healing; it was about embracing a role of service and protection, a commitment to fight for not just my own life, but for the lives of others who were lost in the same darkness I had known. This realization instilled a renewed sense of purpose and direction, fueling my resolve to emerge stronger and more determined than ever.

EMBRACING A NEW REALITY

In the quietude of reflection, a profound understanding dawned upon me: to move forward, I needed to fundamentally reframe my world. This meant confronting and accepting aspects of my new reality that were incredibly difficult to face. Central to this was the necessity of a different kind of surrender, one that involved coming to terms with the most heart-wrenching loss I had experienced.

The hardest part of this process was letting go of my son or, more precisely, the version of him that I knew and loved in this physical world. This wasn't about erasing his memory or diminishing the love I held for him. Rather, it was about acknowledging that while he was no longer physically present, his spirit and the essence of our bond would continue to live within me.

This surrender was not a resignation but a poignant acceptance of our temporary separation in this earthly life. It was a commitment to carry his memory with me, allowing it to inspire and guide me until the day we would be reunited. This acceptance was crucial for me to embrace the life I still had to live—a life that I resolved should be filled with purpose, love, and service to others.

This shift in perspective was a crucial aspect of my journey through grief. It represented a surrender not to despair, but to the transformative power of love and memory. It was about finding a way to continue living a meaningful life, infused with the love and lessons my son left behind. This was the essence of surrender as I came to understand it: a powerful, active choice that paved the way for healing, growth, and the continuation of a life marked by profound love and purpose.

A PARADOXICAL FREEDOM

In our quest for peace amidst profound grief, I've come to understand that all paths ultimately lead us to a pivotal moment of surrender. While this concept often gets entwined with acceptance, the final stage of the conventional grief model, I find "surrender" a more apt term. It implies a more active engagement, a conscious choice made after an arduous journey of internal struggle and emotional upheaval.

Wrestling with life's fiercest challenges, facing metaphorical monsters, shedding countless tears, and laying bare our souls all converge at a point where we are confronted with the unthinkable—accepting what once seemed unacceptable. This isn't about passive resignation but about an empowered yielding.

This might sound counterintuitive at first. Why surrender? Why accept the seemingly unacceptable? Yet, therein lies a paradoxical freedom. The therapies and tools I've spoken of— vision statements, meditation, breathing, and the like—are not mere practices. They are guides, leading us to a place where we can willingly surrender to life's twists and turns. Imagine walking through a dense forest, where each step is laden with uncertainty and pain, and then suddenly, you step into a clearing. This clearing is the space of surrender.

This chapter is an invitation to you, the reader, to explore this clearing for yourself. I hope it will help guide you to this threshold and help you to cross it when you're ready. There's a profound healing that awaits on the other side, a healing that is only accessible when surrender is embraced in its truest form.

Chapter 13:
ENCOURAGING HEALING

Lessons Learned

I n the cool, early hours of a Coronado morning, the world was bathed in the soft hues of dawn, casting a tranquil glow over the quiet beach. Dressed in my lightweight running gear, I savored the solitude and fresh ocean air, a stark contrast to the warm, cozy hotel room where my wife and daughter lay sleeping. This morning ritual, a sacred time carved out of each day, was my commitment to personal goals and self-care. As the sleeping city whispered around me, I set out along the shoreline, my feet finding a steady rhythm on the cool, damp sand, the gentle roar of the ocean waves a constant companion in the quiet of the dawn.

Gasping for breath, my heart pounding fiercely, I pushed through the final stretch of my morning run, the mantra of strength, love, and passion for my family pulsating through my mind.

"Come on, son, let's go! Let's get it!" I urged, imagining Xanny running beside me, sharing in the exertion and exhilaration. As the familiar rock marker came into view, I sprinted with all the energy I had left, crossing that symbolic finish line and feeling the rush of achievement flood through me.

Bent over, hands on knees, I gasped, drawing in deep, satisfying breaths, relishing the joy of meeting my goal. The physical intensity of the run melded with an emotional release, a perfect harmony of body and spirit. Then, almost instinctively, I fell into my breathing routine, the world around me fading as I focused inward: inhale one-two-three, hold, exhale one-two-three, hold. Each count, a whispered cadence, echoing in the rhythm of my heart.

With my eyes closed, I slipped into a meditative trance, my son's voice ringing clear and bright in my ears, "That's a good run, dad, you really pushed yourself today!" I felt the ghostly touch of his hand on my shoulder, a comforting pressure. Turning to embrace him, I found only the open air as I opened my eyes, the illusion shattered, snapping me back to reality.

The stark absence of Xanny hit me anew, a wave of grief rising like a tide, threatening to overwhelm me as it once did. But I stood firm, allowing the sorrow to wash over me, not as a force of destruction but as a testament to the boundless love I held for my son. The grief reached its crest, then ebbed away, replaced by a profound sense of gratitude that welled up from deep within.

Gratitude for Xanny, for my journey, for Debra and for Ava. Gratitude for the myriad blessings in my life, the friends, family, and colleagues whose love and support have been my strength, the opportunities I've had to touch the lives of others and to be touched in return.

Looking out at the ocean, I realized the rhythmic dance of the waves mirrored my own existence—the continuous flow of grief and gratitude, loss and love, reflecting and surrendering. In this eternal dance, joy remains the core, a steadfast promise that one day, when I reunite with Xanny, it will be complete and unending.

***

REASONS TO CONTINUE AND HEAL

As with most things in life, when you look back at your journey through grief, you'll see patterns emerge. From watching the natural rhythm of the ocean for hours on end, the pattern of waves crashing forward then the waters receding, continually ebbing and flowing back and forth, I adapted my own pattern of allowing myself time to continue to grieve over Xan's passing but to then immediately follow that time with gratitude. I repeat this pattern every birthday, angelversary, and Christmas—and at other, unexpected times, too, when needed. It's a healthy part of who I am now, cleansing and natural.

Great love includes great grief. I need these moments of grief and gratitude. It's the ying and the yang, the push and the pull, the sorrow and the joy that allow surrender and acceptance to come forth. Finding your pattern is helpful for allowing grace for yourself and loved ones close to you.

In the depths of grief, it can be hard to find reasons to continue, to push through the pain towards healing. But these reasons exist, sometimes hidden beneath layers of sorrow, waiting to be uncovered and embraced.

One reason to keep moving forward is the people who still need you, who love you and rely on your presence in their lives. As I came to realize, your family, friends, and perhaps even those you have yet to meet, are all threads in the intricate tapestry of your life. Your healing is not just for you; it's for them as well. It's a way of showing up, not just physically, but emotionally and spiritually, for those who are part of your journey.

Another reason lies in the legacy of the loved one you have lost. Carrying their memory forward in a way that honors their impact on your life is a powerful motivator. It's about keeping their spirit alive, not just in your memories, but in your actions and choices. Each step towards healing can be a step towards celebrating their life, making sure that their influence continues to be felt in the world.

There's also a reason that resides within yourself—your own well-being and the fulfillment of your potential. The journey of healing can lead to personal growth, a deeper understanding of yourself, and an increased capacity for empathy and compassion. It can open doors to new perspectives, new relationships, and new experiences.

Ultimately, the most profound reason to continue and to heal is the recognition that life, despite its trials and tribulations, is precious. There is beauty to be found, love to be shared, and joy to be experienced. Your journey through grief is a part of your story, but it doesn't have to be the entire narrative. There is more to your life than your loss, and in that realization lies a powerful reason to seek healing.

THE SPIRITUAL JOURNEY OF HEALING

In my journey through grief and rediscovery, I've found a profound parallel with the principles of Alcoholics Anonymous (AA). Just as those grappling with the despair of addiction often find themselves at the end of their own strength, leading them to the Twelve Steps, so too does the journey through grief often bring us to a point of spiritual dependence and awakening.

Grief, much like addiction, can make us feel utterly powerless, our lives seemingly unmanageable in the face of loss. The Twelve Steps of AA emphasize a turning point: the realization of our own limitations and the decision to turn our will and our lives over to the care of God as we understand Him. This principle is not just vital for overcoming addiction; it is equally crucial in navigating the treacherous waters of grief.

I understand the temptation to distance oneself from God, especially when He seems responsible for the pain and suffering we endure. It's a natural response to want to run as far away as possible from a source we associate with our deepest hurts. But in my experience, this is a mistake. Running away from the source, from God, means facing the monsters of grief and despair alone.

Turning to God, however, opens a different path. It's not an easy path, nor is it a quick solution. It may involve hard questions, nights filled with angry prayers and tears, and the daunting step of reaching out for help, perhaps even walking through church doors for the first time in a long while. But in turning to God, we find strength, knowledge, wisdom, and guidance on our journey to healing.

God's presence in this journey does not immediately dispel all pain or answer all questions. Yet, it provides a foundation of hope and a promise of enduring support. He is there to help you to navigate through the darkest nights, to offer a hand when you stumble, and to listen when you cry out in anger or despair. He is there to help you find the breadcrumbs of hope, to see the signs of His love, and to guide you gently towards healing.

Believe that in turning to God, you are not walking this path alone. He is more than capable of guiding you through to the other side of grief. It's a journey that requires faith, patience, and a willingness to confront the difficult aspects of loss. But with God, this journey can lead to a place of peace, understanding, and a renewed sense of purpose. Remember, in the depths of grief, there is a path to healing, and it starts with looking up, turning to God as you understand Him, and taking that first step toward Him.

EMBRACING A JOURNEY OF ENDLESS HORIZONS

While I draw this book to close, I know my journey to healing has not ended. From the depths of despair to the peaks of understanding, this path has been anything but straightforward. Yet, it's in this intricate dance of loss, grief, and eventual surrender that we find the true essence of healing and growth.

The stories and insights shared in these pages are more than just a recounting of personal experiences; they are a beacon of hope for anyone navigating the turbulent seas of grief. Remember, surrender is not about giving up; it's about opening up to new possibilities of living and loving, even in the face of overwhelming loss.

As you turn the last page of this book, I invite you to see it not as an end, but as a beginning, a starting point for your own journey towards healing and acceptance. The road ahead may still have its twists and turns, its ups and downs, but now you are equipped with the knowledge that even in the darkest times, there is a light that guides us forward.

To you, the reader, navigating your own sea of grief, I extend this message: Do not give up. The journey you are on may feel endless and the pain insurmountable, but there is a path forward. Healing, though it may seem like a distant dream, is within your reach.

I understand the temptation to succumb to despair, to allow the waves of sorrow to pull you under. I've been there, in that dark place where hope seems like a forgotten language. But I urge you to fight against that pull. Your story, like mine, does not end with loss. There is more to be written, more chapters to be lived.

Seeking healing is not a betrayal of your loved one's memory. It is, in fact, a tribute to them. It's a way of honoring the love you shared by continuing to live, to find joy, and to cherish their impact on your life. It's a journey of carrying their legacy forward, not in the shadows of sadness, but in the light of love and remembrance.

I encourage you to take small steps towards healing. These steps might be as simple as talking about your loss, engaging in activities that bring you peace, or seeking support from friends, family, or professionals. Remember, healing is not a linear process. There will be setbacks and difficult days, but each step forward, no matter how small, is progress.

You are not alone in this. There are others who have walked this path and have found a way through. Lean on them, learn from them, and allow their stories to inspire your own journey.

Your grief is unique, but the quest for healing is a shared human experience.

Hold onto the love and memories of those you've lost, for they become the guiding stars in your night sky. Let their legacy be a source of strength and inspiration as you forge a new path, one marked by resilience, hope, and a deeper understanding of life's impermanence.

May you find peace in the knowledge that the journey of grief is not a solitary one. We are all travelers on this path, each with our unique stories and experiences, yet connected by the universal threads of loss and love. In this shared humanity, we find comfort, solidarity, and the courage to move forward.

So, as we conclude, remember that every end is a new beginning. Your story does not end here. It evolves, grows, and continues to unfold in beautiful and unexpected ways. May you embrace this journey with an open heart, knowing that the horizons ahead are endless and filled with potential for joy, fulfillment, and newfound purpose.

Thank you for walking this path with me. May your journey ahead be one of healing, discovery, and profound peace.

EPILOGUE

Health Check

The day I lost my son marked the most tragic day of my life. Since then, I've spent countless hours, days, and weeks, both voluntarily and involuntarily, analyzing every moment leading up to that fateful day and every day since, seeking a path through the dark forest of grief.

I want to take a brief moment to speak to you from my heart. There are moments in life when we must pause and scrutinize our circumstances. Your experience may mirror mine, grappling with the overwhelming loss of a loved one. Or, perhaps you're navigating the aftermath of a divorce, the dissolution of a dream, the repercussions of a life-altering accident, or the enduring scars of childhood traumas. Whether you're enveloped in depression, ensnared by daily anxiety, or paralyzed by fear, I want to offer you a glimmer of hope: healing is attainable.

I implore you to consider your own situation. Are you in danger? Is your heart, mind, or spirit signaling a crisis you've yet to confront? You don't have to wait for your world to crumble before making life-saving changes for yourself or your loved ones. Take a moment to ponder these questions: Are there warning signs in my life that I'm overlooking or inadequately addressing? Am I in the midst of an emergency that could alter the course of my life? Is it time for drastic action?

Take a moment with me now to take stock of your current place, just a brief moment right here and now, and reflect with me. Ask yourself these questions:

Question 1: Are there warning signs?

Are there warning signs in my life that I am overlooking or inadequately addressing? It's not uncommon to feel guilt or believe that certain situations are unchangeable, leading to resignation and continued suffering. But ignoring problems only brings temporary relief. Confronting the truth, though painful, is necessary. Acknowledging these signs, jotting them down, and piecing together a comprehensive picture is crucial.

Question 2: Am I in an emergency?

Am I in the midst of an emergency that could alter the course of my life? It's possible to be in a dire situation without recognizing it, especially if it has become your norm. You might be accustomed to thoughts of giving up, fear for a loved one's safety, or feelings of hitting rock bottom. Mental and emotional struggles can blind you to the reality of your situation, making you feel like you're already at your worst when, in truth, you might be teetering on the edge of a life-or-death situation. I don't want you to wait any longer if you find yourself in such a situation.

Question 3: Is it time for drastic measures?

Is it time for an intervention or drastic action? If I could turn back time, I would have stopped everything for my son. I thought we were doing enough at the time, but that drive to Flagstaff changed everything. I realized I was willing, wishing, wanting to do so much more. I was prepared to pull him out of school, take a leave of absence, or even quit my job—whatever it took to keep him safe. If you're sensing these warning signs, if you feel that you're in an emergency, don't hesitate. The alternative is a reality from which you cannot return.

If you need immediate help, please refer to the resources here. You might need to reach out to family, friends, authorities, or helplines for support. You may need to take a first step. If that's you, please don't wait.

Remember, you are not alone in this.

If you find yourself in an emergency, act now! There's no shame in seeking aid. Your life is precious, and as long as you draw breath, you have a purpose. God is not finished with you.

EMERGENCY RESOURCES

1. National Suicide Prevention Lifeline (United States)

    - Phone: 1-800-273-TALK (1-800-273-8255)

    - Online Chat: https://suicidepreventionlifeline.org/chat/

    - Offers free, 24/7 confidential support for people in distress

2. Crisis Text Line

    - Text "HELLO" to 741741 (United States)

    - Offers 24/7 support via text with trained crisis counselors

3. Emergency Services

    - Phone: 911 (United States) or your country's emergency service number

    - For immediate assistance in life-threatening situations

Interventional and Support Resources

1. Substance Abuse and Mental Health Services Administration (SAMHSA)

    - Phone: 1-800-662-HELP (1-800-662-4357)

    - Offers general information on mental health and can help locate local treatment services

2. National Alliance on Mental Illness (NAMI)

    - Helpline: 1-800-950-NAMI (1-800-950-6264)

    - Provides support, information, and referrals for mental health concerns

3. BetterHelp
   - Website: https://www.betterhelp.com
   - Offers access to licensed therapists for online counseling and therapy

4. Talkspace
   - Website: https://www.talkspace.com/
   - Provides online therapy with licensed therapists

5. GriefShare
   - Website: https://www.griefshare.org/
   - A network of support groups for people grieving the loss of a loved one

6. DivorceCare
   - Website: https://www.divorcecare.org/
   - Support groups for those going through separation or divorce

7. Alcoholics Anonymous (AA)
   - Website: https://www.aa.org/
   - A fellowship of individuals who share their experience with alcoholism and help others to recover

8. National Domestic Violence Hotline
   - Phone: 1-800-799-SAFE (1-800-799-7233)
   - Provides 24/7 crisis intervention, safety planning, and information on domestic violence

General Mental Health and Wellness Resources

1. Substance Abuse and Mental Health Services Administration

   - Website: https://www.mentalhealth.gov/
   - Provides information on mental health disorders and resources for support

2. Psychology Today Therapist Finder

   - Website: https://www.psychologytoday.com/us/therapists
   - A tool to find therapists in your area based on your specific needs

3. Xan You Matter Foundation

   - Website: https://www.xanyoumatter.org
   - Our organization to help break the stigma around mental health. The Xan You Matter Foundation is dedicated to providing support and resources for individuals facing depression, anxiety, and suicidal ideation, striving to bring hope and end the stigma around mental health.

Note:

The resources provided below are intended to offer immediate assistance and support. Given the dynamic nature of online information, names and organizations may change over time. If you encounter difficulty accessing the listed resources, we recommend searching for the organization's name or helpline number using an internet search engine like Google. By entering the organization's name or helpline number into the search bar, you can locate the most up-to-date contact information and access their services effectively.

Remember, seeking help is a sign of strength, not weakness.

-Ignacio E. Leon

ABOUT THE AUTHOR

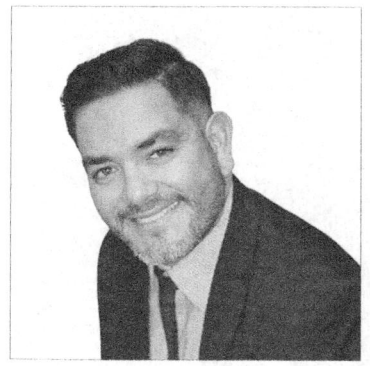

Ignacio E. Leon has traversed an extraordinary path from a high-level executive in the financial sector to an example of hope and transformation in the realm of mental health advocacy. As the driving force behind Make Shift Happen and the co-founder and vice president of the Xan You Matter Foundation with his wife, Debra, his life's work is dedicated to fostering resilience and offering solace to those grappling with grief.

A seasoned professional, Ignacio's acumen in business management and strategic development was honed through years of leadership, overseeing teams and spearheading initiatives that propelled corporate success. His academic pursuits, culminating in advanced degrees, underpin a career marked by determination and a commitment to excellence.

Yet, it was the personal upheaval following the loss of his son, Alexander Estefan Leon, that steered Ignacio towards a deeper, more introspective journey. This pivotal moment birthed "Rising from the Ashes," a book that not only tells his story but also serves as a guide for others navigating the pain of loss, encapsulating his belief in the transformative power of resilience.

Today, Ignacio resides in Phoenix, Arizona, with his wife and daughter, surrounded by a close-knit community of friends and family. His life in Phoenix is a testament to the healing and growth that can emerge from life's trials, reflecting the very essence of his advocacy and work. Through his speaking, writing, and community engagement, Ignacio continues to inspire and support individuals in their quest for healing and transformation.

For more information on Ignacio's journey, his initiatives, and the impact of his work, visit www.makeshifthappennow.com

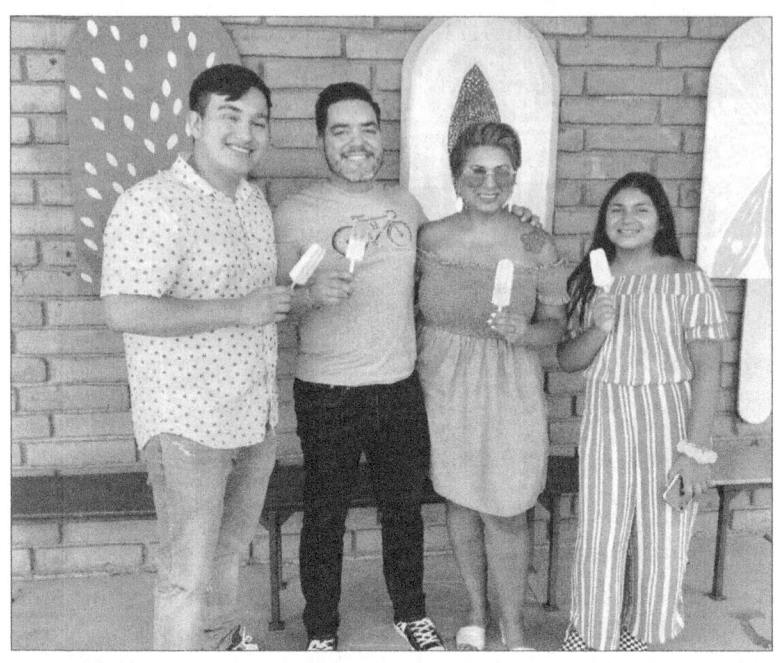

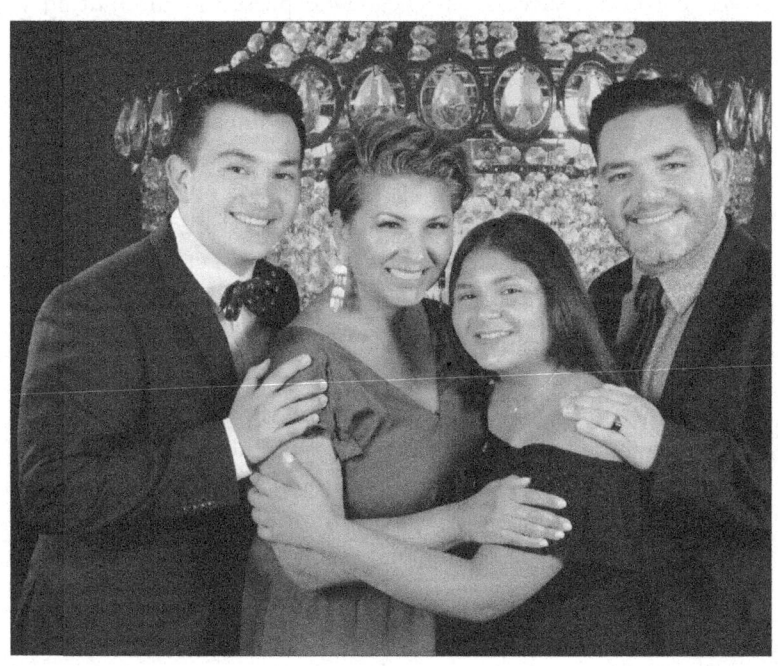

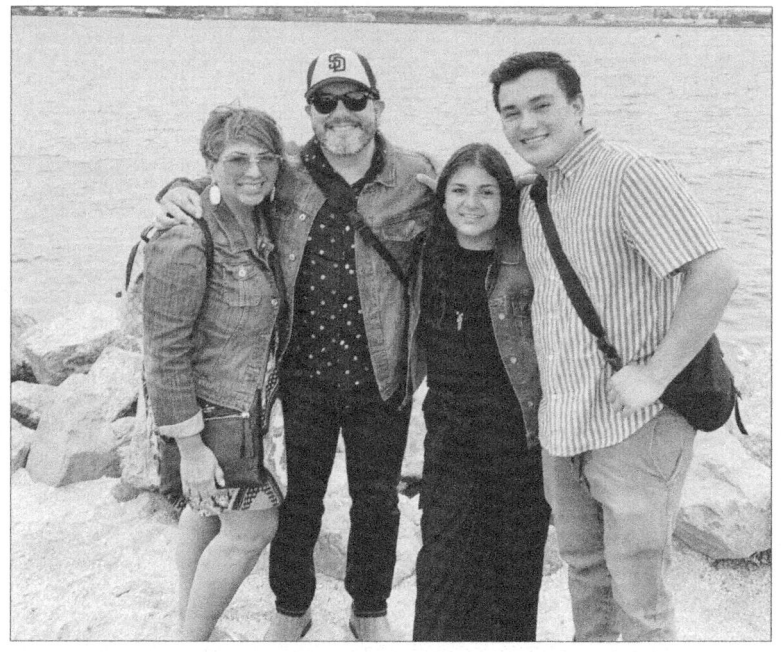

Made in United States
North Haven, CT
20 October 2024

59183311R10078